Gabriel Asulin

Turn your Dental Practice into a Successful Business

The Gabriel Asulin Method

Gabriel Asulin
Turn your Dental Practice into a Successful Business
The Gabriel Asulin Method

Translation from Hebrew: Shira Levy
Grammatical Editing: Polina Brill

Cover Design: Studio Medico

© All rights reserved to the author
Printed by Zameret Books

Printed in Israel 2018

ISBN 9781731511973

Without limiting the rights under copyright reserved above, no part of the publication may be reproduce, stored into a retrieval system, or transmitted, in any from or by any mean (electric, mechanical, photocopying, recording, or otherwise), Without the prior written permission of the author.

www.dentalmarketing.co.il

Contents

Introduction 5

PART ONE: DENTAL PRACTICE MARKETING. 7

Chapter 1 – How Do Clients Choose a Practice? 9

Chapter 2 – The Complex Marketing of the Dental Practice 12

Chapter 3 – Retaining Customers 15

Chapter 4 – Positioning and Differentiation 28

PART TWO: BUSINESS POLICY AND MANAGEMENT OF PRACTICE STAFF 35

Chapter 5 – Receptionist Conduct 37

Chapter 6 – Rewarding and Increasing Staff Motivation 59

Chapter 7 – "Personal Branding" of Dentists 67

Chapter 8 – Assistants' Conduct with the Dentist and Clients 74

Chapter 9 – The Dental Hygienist's Conduct and Increased Productivity 77

Chapter 10 – Pricing Strategy for Treatments 82

PART THREE: THE ART OF CLOSING TREATMENT PLANS 87

Chapter 11 – The Dentist's Self-Marketing when Meeting with Clients 89

Chapter 12 – Closing Treatment Plans 101

PART FOUR: ATTRACTING NEW CLIENTS TO THE PRACTICE . . 137

Chapter 13 – How to Attract New Clients to the Practice 139

PART FIVE: THE PRACTICE'S BUSINESS CONDUCT 157

Chapter 14 – Realizing the Practice's Potential. 159

Chapter 15 – Recommended Business Strategy 161

Chapter 16 – The Practice's Financial Conduct. 164

Chapter 17 – Opening a New Dental Practice or Relocating 167

Chapter 18 – Dealing with Competitors 179

Chapter 19 – Aesthetic Treatments 181

PART SIX: MISCELLANEOUS 185

Chapter 20 – Dealing with Demanding Customers 187

Chapter 21 – Business Conduct during the Holidays 190

Chapter 22 – The Little Things that Make a Big Difference 192

Your Practice Can Earn More! 195

Introduction

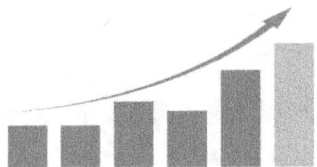

Growing competition in the dental industry has created new rules for the game: it is no longer enough to be a professional dentist in order to succeed financially.

Today marketing, promotion, and effective management of a practice are essential conditions for its existence and success. A dental practice is a business like any other, and as you will discover in this book, management and marketing are complex matters that include a wide variety of aspects. These aspects need to be applied in order to make your dental practice successful financially.

The new and updated management and marketing tactics which I offer in this new and expanded edition of the book **How to Turn your Dental Practice into a Successful Business** are based on experience in consulting and business support for hundreds of dental practices around the world. These methods have been successfully applied in many dental practices, and have proven to significantly improve sale cycles and profitability.

The vast experience I have accumulated over the years proves that any practice can improve its sale cycles by tens of percent and even more. All it takes is to pause for a moment, objectively examine the methods used by the practice, and be open to adopting new and more effective management and marketing tactics. Sometimes it is enough to improve just one or two parameters when managing and marketing the practice in order to see a significant improvement its performance and profit.

I suggest that you not only read this book but also apply what you read in order to improve your practice's bottom line.

Here's to pleasant and helpful reading,
Gabriel Asulin

PART ONE

DENTAL PRACTICE MARKETING

Chapter 1

How Do Clients Choose a Practice?

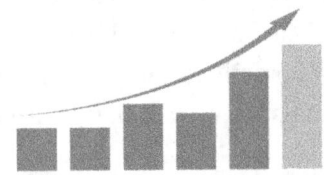

The million-dollar question in dental practice marketing is, How do customers decide on a practice in which to receive care? Although going to the dentist is not something people look forward to, at some point clients must decide on a dentist or practice. As professionals, it is important that we understand the customers' decision-making process, because if we know what is important to them and understand how they make decisions, we can make the necessary adjustments so that they will ultimately turn to us for dental care.

In the context of consumer behavior, one of the most popular models which attempts to explain consumer decision-making processes is the Fishbein Model. According to the Fishbein Model, when a customer faces a complex purchasing decision, he or she will execute a market survey and examine, on average, three alternatives. During the market survey, the customer will formulate a position that constitutes a "score" for each alternative examined. This is done based on the parameters they find most important, such as quality of care, costs, etc. According to this model, the brand that receives the highest weighted score among the alternatives examined will be chosen. For example, a student will choose a car that receives the highest score in the categories of savings and reliability, since these parameters are most important to him or her. A wealthy family man, on the other hand, will choose the safest and most spacious car. How, then, will Mr. Smith choose a dentist or dental practice according to the Fishbein Model? The answer is – in approximately the same way.

First, we must answer two important questions: What are the most important parameters when choosing a dentist or dental practice? And, how much weight do customers attribute to each parameter?

During my first years as a dental practice consultant, I made sure to conduct market surveys in each practice I worked with – partly because I wanted to identify the specific strengths and weaknesses of each practice, but also in order to learn about how consumers of dental care thought.

One of my questions in the internal and external surveys was, what do you consider the most important features when choosing a dental practice? The results did not surprise me, but they did surprise many practice owners. What did surprise me was the fact that the results were almost identical across all the practices. The process of choosing a dentist or dental practice is, in fact, the same pretty much everywhere even though many professionals are certain that their location has its own rules.

Let us review the results – the four most important features for dental customers, in order of importance:
1. Professionalism of the dentist or dental practice
2. Personal attention
3. The practice's location
4. Treatment prices

You're probably not surprised by these, but we should pay attention to the importance attributed by customers to every category: The dentist or practice's professionalism is the most important parameter and impacts 53% of the customer's decision. Personal attention is the second most important parameter and affects about 31% of the customer's decision. The location of the practice is the third most important parameter and constitutes about 9% of the customer's decision. Last on this list is the price, surprisingly. The parameter that we might have guessed would be the most important constitutes only about 7% of the client's decision when choosing a dentist or dental practice.

Incidentally, additional studies show almost identical results. A survey conducted by the Zimmer Implant Company, which examined patients who underwent or were meant to undergo dental implant surgery, found that the price of the implant surgery was the last parameter in the clients' list of considerations and affected only 4% of customer decisions. In fact, the longevity of the implant, which is in fact the "professionalism," was shown to carry the most weight among customers: 55%.

Simply put, customers give you and your practice a total score based on the qualities that are most important to them and compare these scores with the scores of the other practices. If you receive the highest score, the customer will decide to undergo treatments at your practice. If your competitor receives a higher score than you do, the customer will turn to them for dental care.

The most interesting fact is that the practice's professionalism (53%) and personal attention (31%) constitute a whopping 84% of clients' decision process when choosing a dentist or practice. Therefore, it is reasonable to assume that whoever wins when it comes to these two parameters will win the customers over. If we narrow down the reasons for winning the customer's heart and pocket, we can say that most practices have a relatively good score in the field of personal attention (I have encountered only a few cases of practices that severely mistreat their clients) and therefore those who succeed in producing the best professional impression win the client over.

It is worth noting that these considerations are the average, and apply to most customers; however, there are customers who put different weight on different parameters. There are, for example, those who are so afraid of the dentist that the parameter of personal attention and empathy exhibited by the dentist are most important to them. There are also some for whom price is most important. These patients convince themselves that there are no differences between practices, or even if they prefer another option, they can't afford the price. However, as the surveys I conducted show, for the vast majority of customers professionalism and personal attention are the most important in choosing a dentist or practice.

Many dentists mistakenly believe that customers prefer their competitors because they offer lower prices. It's always easier to blame the price than to admit that you failed at the sales process.

Customers who prefer a competitor whose prices are lower do so, in most cases, not because of the price but rather because the more expensive practice was unable to show them that it was also more professional and that there is justification for the higher prices it charges.

Remember – customers are willing to pay more (within reason) on the condition that they understand the additional benefits they will receive for the higher prices. This is basic consumer behavior. It is no accident that the bestselling vehicle worldwide in recent years is the Toyota. Consumers believe that they get more for their money – reliability, saving, value, etc., and are therefore willing to pay more.

Chapter 2

The Complex Marketing of the Dental Practice

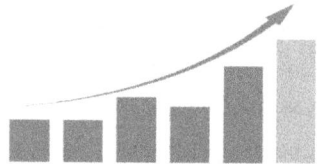

In order to perform internal or external marketing for the dental practice effectively, the differences between marketing a service and marketing a product must be understood and internalized. Many academic books deal with the complexity of marketing the services of professionals and with the nuances of formulating a service marketing strategy. One point is overwhelmingly agreed upon: it is easier to market toothpaste than it is to market dental care. The main reason for this is the essential difference between a product and a service. The product is tangible, as opposed to the service, which is intangible. This data makes the purchase decision made by the clients, when coming to "buy" dentistry, very complex.

Note the differences between purchasing a product versus a service in the following example. Mr. Smith wants to buy a car. Before he makes the decision, he has the option to check out the car at a professional institute and take a test drive so that he can get a feel for the car and assess the strength of the engine. He also has accurate data on car quality: engine volume, horsepower, precise fuel consumption, etc. Moreover, he receives a warranty. Thus, Mr. Smith, when making the purchase, is in a state of almost complete certainty regarding how much he is paying and what he is getting in return.

However, when Mr. Smith comes to a dental practice, his decision-making process is fundamentally different and he finds himself in an almost absurd situation. He needs to be in the position to say, "I'm willing to pay X amount, and to put my dental care in Dr. Y's hands" – and this before he has anything in hand. Moreover, he will actually never know what he got, even at the end of the treatment. After all, he has no way of knowing whether the implants lasted only four years because of the dentist's sub-par work, the quality of the implants themselves, or gum problems. He will never have an answer to the question, "If I had gone to Dr. Jones instead, would the implants have lasted longer?"

Another point that only increases uncertainty in customers is the fact that they have no idea what exactly the dentist is doing in their mouth. Therefore, they have no way of measuring the dentist's professionalism and the quality of care they receive. The only thing they can measure is whether the injection was painful.

To go back to the absurdity of the purchase decision in the field of dentistry, a customer is supposed to say "Yes!" to a treatment plan at a very high cost before they even know what they will receive, whether Dr. X will perform the best treatment, whether the treatment plan is the best plan for them, or how long the treatment will be. If this isn't absurd, what is?

These are your customers and this is how they feel: confused, uncertain, in a difficult decision-making position, nervous (who wouldn't be?), and at times – they are annoying. The reality is, those who step into their shoes and understand how they feel and act, will win them over.

Even though clients are helpless regarding the final return on their payment and have no tools with which to measure the dentist's professionalism, they know that their teeth need care and have no choice but to decide at which practice to receive that care. If so, how do clients, surrounded by uncertainty, still decide which practice to turn to? How can they assess who is a professional dentist, even though they have no idea what the dentist is actually doing?

The answer is simple, though cruel. Because, as mentioned above, clients do not have the ability to assess the quality of the practice and dentist's professionalism, they will judge you according to your conduct. In other words, customers will be able to assess if you are professional through the elements they encounter when visiting the practice.

New clients, when entering a practice for the first time, activate all of their senses in order to determine, "Have I come to the right place?" Clients operate using the Mosaic Method: they collect some data and build a quick positive or negative first impression about the practice. Incidentally, building the first impression mosaic takes no more than 40 seconds. Marketing experts claim that it is at this point that customers decide, in principle, whether or not they want to be attached to the business. Notice what happens when we enter a restaurant for the first time; surely you too have left after a few seconds. A dirty fork or a strange smell is enough to build a negative first impression and disqualify the business.

Potential clients will start building the mosaic when they call the practice for the first time – and judge how long it took for the phone to be answered, how they were spoken to, and so on. In later stages, they will judge the practice according to the following criteria: Did the appointment begin on time? Did the receptionist smile and offer them a drink? Was the practice clean? Were other customers waiting in line or arguing with the receptionist?

I did warn you that this was a cruel matter – if clients encounter the wrong conduct, they will come to the simple conclusion that this practice is unprofessional. Clients cannot measure what is being done in their mouths, but they can measure the team's behavior and, based on this, decide whether the practice is professional. Objectively this is not the right way to judge a practice, but this is the reality. When you think about it, this is the only option available to potential customers.

Let me tell you a story. A dentist invited me to examine his dental practice. "Many customers come to me for examinations, but only a small percentage of them remain and undergo treatments," he told me anxiously, as we sat in the practice's waiting room. In front of us stood a filthy aquarium full of green water and two poor fish; it was unclear how they had managed to survive. The smell in the practice was unpleasant; the lighting and the furniture were from the era of World War II. If that was not enough, the dentist was wearing a stained uniform that looked at least a decade old.

I summed up the consumer behavior theory and probably the reason for the problem he invited me to solve: "If this is the way your aquarium looks, your work is unprofessional." Paradoxically, this was a specialist, a graduate of a prestigious dental school, and seemed to be doing a better job than many of his competitors. However, as I mentioned, because clients do not have the tools with which to measure his functional professionalism, they judge him based on subjective characteristics: the unpleasant smell in the practice and the dirty aquarium.

Chapter 3

Retaining Customers

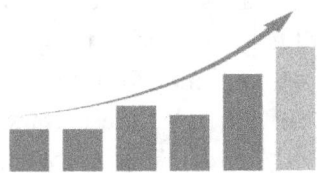

The most important parameter for the success of a dental practice as a business entity is, undoubtedly, customer loyalty. A practice that has succeeded in gaining highly loyal customers will gain significant customer intake and hence business success. On the other hand, a practice in which only a small percentage of customers show loyalty will not survive for long. In fact, loyal customers are considered the engine that drives any business, and certainly when it comes to a dental practice. Why? Because loyal customers have the following three characteristics, without which no business or practice can survive for long.

1. Returning customers: Loyal customers who do not switch dentists or practices and remain loyal for a long time, even if the practice moves to another location (at a reasonable distance). In this context, it should be noted that customers suffering from "dentist anxiety" would continue to be loyal to their dentist from the moment they find a dentist who has won their trust, even if the dentist moves many kilometers away. By the way, this is not a small market – data indicates that about 30% of the public reports some type of dental anxiety.

2. "Ambassador" clients: These clients are sure to tell their acquaintances about the practice and recommend that they receive care there and only there. Studies show that satisfied customers pass on recommendations to about four consumers, as opposed to unsatisfied customers, who tell 12 people about their experience. "Ambassador" customers contribute to the success of the practice relatively more than businesses in other areas for the simple reason that in most cases, a client who approaches your practice, especially when it comes to complex and expensive dental treatments, has already consulted with one of your existing clients.

3. **"Price insensitive" clients**: Loyal clients who are not price-sensitive, as compared with disloyal ones. When a brand satisfies the client's wishes, they will continue to purchase their products, even if they are more expensive than the alternatives (within reason). The same applies to your loyal customers – if they show loyalty to you, you probably gave them a good reason to do so, and they will remain loyal to you even if the competition offers less expensive treatments.

There is only one small problem: studies have shown that customer loyalty is declining. Until the mid-1980s, people in some countries outside of the United States drove a certain type of car, smoked a certain type of local cigarette, and drank one particular type of coffee. Today these brands are in danger of extinction; consumers prefer American cigarettes, they discovered the taste of the granulated instant coffee that comes in attractive glass packages and the coffee capsules of the home coffee machines, and they prefer to drive Japanese cars. The erosion of consumer loyalty to a specific brand is a global phenomenon that threatens every business and organization. The erosion of loyalty is the present, and forgive my pessimism, but all the signs point to the continuation of this trend.

Another no less significant reason for declining loyalty is the intensity of competition. In the past fifteen years, the number of dentists in some places has doubled, and as of today, the ratio of dentists per capita in certain countries is considered one the highest there has ever been. When customers are offered a greater number of alternatives they feel more courted, more exposed to temptations and offers; as competition grows, their bargaining power grows accordingly. I'm not sure that this is comforting, but the drastic rise in the intensity of competition did not skip over anyone in the business world.

Are your practice's customers loyal to you? Chances are that only a small percentage of them are. If we count the number of customers who have put their mouths in your hands over the past ten years, and check how many of them have also remained active at the practice, we will probably discover a large percentage of customers who have "evaporated."

What Leads Clients to Develop Loyalty or Disloyalty to a Practice?

Many consumer behavior studies have been conducted in order to try to crack the DNA of customer loyalty. In fact, the question of customer loyalty is what interests most of the marketing world in the 21st century. Everyone knows how to bring in new customers: advertise and advertise (and spend a lot of money). But how the heck do we make customers stay loyal and recommend the practice to their acquaintances? This is more complicated.

All studies and models of customer loyalty can be summarized in one simple, logical equation: The more satisfied customers are with the return on their money, the higher the level of loyalty to the practice they will develop, and vice versa. By the way, satisfaction arises when customers feel that their expectations have been met and that they received a full return on their investment – "I paid 100 and got 100 in return."

If that's so, the question arises: If satisfaction is the most influential factor in loyalty then why don't most customers develop loyalty to the dental practice? Was the practice unable to satisfy them and give them full value for their money? An interesting and comprehensive study conducted in recent years by Professor Jacob Hornik from Tel Aviv University and his American colleague, Professor Philip Kotler, provides the answer: The customer's satisfaction, i.e., realizing their expectations and receiving a full return on their investment is no longer enough to build loyalty towards the company. Why? Because customers are over-indulged, spoiled, and demanding nowadays, and see satisfaction as a basic starting point for the purpose of communication but not beyond.

These results are not surprising: today's consumers perceive companies as commercial entities whose main concern is financial gain. As far as customers are concerned, engagement with the company is on a strictly financial basis, and they do not feel any emotional obligation to purchase its products the next time around. "I paid for what I got," the client thinks. "The practice was lucky I turned to them. I don't owe the practice anything; the practice does not owe me. I may come back but don't take me at my word. Thank you very much and good-bye!"

So what about the quality of treatment? You'll be surprised, but they do not really know how to quantify the quality of treatment they received. And as though that were not enough, they know that many other dentists know how to do the same work (unless you're talking about a specialist who performs specific treatments). There is also good news: Hornik and Kotler's study showed that customers who have been "charmed" by a company developed greater loyalty in comparison to customers who have only experienced satisfaction. The study found that over time, charmed customers buy more of the company's products, recommend it to more of their acquaintances, and are less sensitive to that company's prices. If so, who is a "charmed client"? These customers receive more than they expected. In other words, the customer expected to receive 100% in return for their money, but they feel that they received 110%.

In order to focus on the dynamics and effect of charming a client, I will illustrate the matter using another field. Mr. Smith is driving his car and hears a strange noise from the engine. Without thinking twice, he goes to his garage. The mechanic welcomes him, asks how he is and inquiries about his son, opens the hood, makes a few adjustments, and the noise is gone. Mr. Smith thanks the mechanic and asks, "How much do I owe you?" The mechanic answers, "Nothing at all. Have a safe drive."

In this moment, Mr. Smith has been charmed. He expected to pay but the mechanic waived the payment and sent him on his way. Let's think about what happens to Mr. Smith's loyalty to this mechanic for a moment. You can be sure that he will become a loyal customer because one, there is no chance in the world that the next repair will be performed by another garage, two, he plans to recommend the garage to his acquaintances, and three, he won't try to bargain with that mechanic after the next repair.

This will increase customers' loyalty and help retain them:

Everyone wants new customers. Not ten minutes go by after entering a dental practice for the first time before the owner asks me, "How do you bring new clients to the practice?" My usual answer is, "Recruiting new clients is not the problem, actually. The problem is how to keep them."

Here are two interesting facts in this context: First, studies show that the cost of recruiting a new customer is five times higher than the cost of maintaining existing customers. Second, the chance of bringing in a former customer is three times higher than gaining a new one.

Now for the explanation: the cost of recruiting a new customer is five times higher than the cost of retaining an existing customer because acquiring a new customer usually involves considerable financial expenses such as online advertising, ads in the local press, and direct mail campaigns. However, the cost of maintaining existing customers are usually much lower and include minimum expenses only, such as direct mail, e-mail, telephone, and so on.

In addition, the odds of an old customer returning are three times higher than the chances of recruiting a new customer because it is easier for customers to return to something they already know than to turn to something new and unknown. If customers have already been treated by you in the past, it means that you have something they like and if they received good service, you'll probably be able to get them back into the practice.

If this is the case, a practice should first ensure that its existing customers are maintained, and only then turn to the more expensive process of recruiting new ones. It's worthwhile to remember that an average practice, which has existed for several years, has already "hosted" thousands of customers. Therefore, if the practice manages to retain them they will not only use its services, but more importantly, they will be the largest and most significant tool for recruiting new customers. After all, anyone who practices dentistry knows that most new customers come from referrals and not from the local business directory, and as already mentioned in the previous chapters, a satisfied customer recommends his experience to four acquaintances on average.

I know of practices that are more than twenty years old but whose appointment book is empty. Where are the thousands of customers who visited the practice over the years, and by extension, their acquaintances? They need dental care; it's just that they undergo treatment elsewhere.

So why don't customers return? Probably for the simple reason that the practice did not do enough to retain them, so they are likely to have lost any attachment to the practice. When they need dental care, they receive a recommendation for another practice and turn to them instead. It's like staying in touch with friends – you have good friends from school and other periods of life, but after you haven't been in touch for a long time, the friendship dissolves and evaporates. That's exactly what happens with your practice's clients.

Paradoxically, customer retention is not complex; it's actually simple – it is just important to understand its significance instead of blaming customers for their lack of loyalty, and put it at the top of the practice's priority list.

How is this done? Below are five guidelines for increasing customers' loyalty and retaining them as patients.

1. **"Charming" the client** – As noted, studies show that there is a direct relationship between the level of customer satisfaction and the level of loyalty to a product or service. The more you succeed in charming them, the more they will be loyal and recommend the practice to their acquaintances. How do you do this? Very simple: give them more than they expect. Do they expect to get a good return for their money? Give them something beyond that. Here are some examples of how to charm your practice's customers.

   A. **"I just wanted to ask how you are"** - Make a habit of calling customers who visited your practice that day and underwent painful or invasive treatment in order to ask how they are doing. Imagine what happens when a customer is sitting at home in the evening when he suddenly receives a phone call from the dentist or the receptionist and hears, "Hello Mr. Smith, how are you? I just called to make sure that you are doing okay. Is the area still swollen? Don't worry; this is natural after an extraction. Continue with the painkillers and within a day or two the swelling should pass. In any case, if you have any questions please feel free to call us." It is advisable to call not only those who have undergone difficult surgical procedures such as implantations and sinus elevations but anyone who received an injection during treatment. This is a great way to communicate, *We are concerned about your health and well-being, not just your money.* Practices that apply this method tell me that customers are charmed by the phone call they received.

   B. **Charming behavior** – There are many points of contact where you can charm a customer if you internalize the concept that you can give customers more than they expected to receive. For example, a client who asks the receptionist to check on a particular matter and expects an answer only the following day may become charmed if the receptionist calls him only half an hour later and gives him an answer.

   Even trivial matters like offering coffee or remembering the names of the customer's children or an upcoming wedding in the family – these can be recorded in the client's file – may charm them and make them feel wonderful. I know a charming dental practice that records the way clients drink their coffee or tea. When the client sits down in the waiting room the receptionist turns to them after reviewing their file and says, "Mr. Smith, a strong coffee with two sugars, correct?" Believe me, there is no better feeling for a customer.

2. **Stay in touch!** The more time that passes without any contact with the customers, the more the level of their loyalty decreases, just as in personal relationships. Therefore, it is very worthwhile to build a wide range of contact opportunities with the practice's clients, on an annual basis, for example sending a message for the client's birthday or a holiday.

These activities are simple and involve minimal costs; all you have to do is ask your customers for their e-mail address (start now!) and perform all these actions with a click of the mouse. Once you've put together a reasonable number of customer email addresses, you can also send them a monthly or bi-monthly professional article on dentistry – on topics like "Why is it important to brush your tongue too?" or "Are toothpicks harmful to teeth?" and other articles on light and interesting topics.

The expenses involved in performing such activities are insignificant compared to the benefits. Actions of this type will remind clients that the practice exists. Additionally, people really appreciate the fact that they are thought of and remembered after they have paid, not just beforehand.

3. **Periodic checkups: RE-CALLS** – The practice not only needs customers to remember it but also to visit it once every six months. Therefore, periodic checkups are undoubtedly one of the most important aspects of customer retention. Furthermore, RE-CALLS are considered the most effective marketing tool for a dental practice, and it is no wonder – this is a fast, focused marketing tool at a very low cost. Why? Because customers who come in for periodic checkups remain loyal and serve as "ambassadors" for the practice. Moreover, a periodic examination often reveals that they must complete treatments that they have not finished, or require new treatments. Additionally, the checkup includes a dental hygienist, fluorine treatment, and x-rays, and these are also a significant source of income for the practice. Note that the correct terminology is "checkup" rather than "review." Customers perceive "periodic reviews" as being unnecessary, while a "checkup" is perceived as being more important.

The dentist must emphasize the importance of the periodic checkup and even make it a condition of handling the customer's business. It is best for every practice to focus on those who have not visited for over six months. Remember: the more time that has passed since the customer's last visit, the smaller the chances of his or her return and vice versa. On a strategic level, it is better to work with clients who have not visited the practice for a period of six months to two years. You do not have to give up on those who have not been to the practice for the past two years or more. The chances of them returning to the practice are lower, but what can you lose by trying?

So how do you do this most effectively? First, for each customer who has completed treatment, an appointment must be made for six months in the future for a routine checkup. Second, it is important to pay attention to the wording of the appeal. Instead of, "Mr. Smith, you haven't been here for a while, you're invited for a checkup," the following wording should be used: **"Mr. Smith, Dr. Jones has gone over your medical file and asked that we call you up to see whether everything was alright and schedule a checkup. When would this be convenient for you – in the morning or in the evening?"**

Pay attention to the nuances. First, "Dr. Jones asked" gives the customer the feeling that the dentist thinks about him personally. Second, it is a "checkup" rather than a review. Third, "to see that everything is alright"; a client that tells the receptionist that everything is okay and there is no need for a checkup should receive the following answer: "Mr. Smith, you have undergone expensive and complex care. Medically, such treatments must be followed up. If something is wrong it's best to catch it early on to find a quick solution rather than wait until it is too late." Very few customers will dismiss such an appeal.

A final and important point without which RE-CALLS will not be effective is who carries them out and when. In an absolute majority of practices, this is done by the receptionist during the workday and this is where the problems begin. Suppose there is a shift full of emergencies and delays and the receptionist called Bob and invited him for a periodic checkup; Bob was not in front of his calendar and asked the receptionist to call him later. Of course, this conversation will be missed on that day, and Bob will probably not end up having a checkup scheduled for him.

Telemarketing is a Sisyphean task and in order to succeed, it demands a lot of patience, tenacity, and focus. Telemarketers encounter answering machines, unavailable clients, clients who are in an area without reception, clients who cannot speak at that moment, clients who are just boarding a plane on the way to a vacation, or clients who ask to be called the following week. Therefore, receptionists cannot successfully preform telemarketing work in the middle of a shift – not because they are lazy or unmotivated, but because it is impossible to do such work while also receiving payments, booking appointments, and other more urgent responsibilities.

In practice, in the vast majority of practices the receptionist conducts telemarketing work in the middle of the shift. The result? Customers, who answer the phone and are having trouble with their teeth just then, or those highly aware of the importance of periodic checkups, are happy about the call and make an appointment. However, all those who were difficult to reach or need encouragement to make an appointment for checkups in the first place fall between the cracks, do not come for checkups, and at the end of the day disappear from the practice's database. That's why so many established practices, which have seen thousands of customers, have so few periodic checkups and employ a dental hygienist for a shift and a half a week.

It is very important to note that RE-CALLS are one of the best and most important sources of income for a practice. The reason for this is that those who come in for periodic checkups often need treatment ("Mr. Smith, it's time to change that brace; it has run its course"), and they are active customers who serve as "ambassadors" for the practice. However, in order for this to happen, they must first visit the practice, and periodic checkups are the best way to bring them in.

In the United States, the subject of RE-CALLS is highly developed; periodic checkups and work done by a dental hygienist are the main source of income for dental practices. In other countries, on the other hand, many practices dream about attracting new customers and neglect the retention of existing ones. This is with the exception of a small percentage of practices that work correctly, mainly periodontal practices, which produce relatively high outputs of periodic checkups and dental work.

Paradoxically, the way to reach an effective customer retention system for the practice is by way of a large number of periodic checkups and many full shifts for the dental hygienist. It's not only easy it's also cheap – recruiting a telemarketer for a part-time position who will focus exclusively on RE-CALLS will lead to clients streaming into the practice.

The telemarketer should dig into the practice's customer database and find those who have not been to the practice in the past six months or more, and call them in for an examination. I can tell you from experience that the results produced by a dedicated telemarketer can be amazing. Of course, part of the database may no longer be relevant (customers who have moved away, for example), but what can you lose by picking up a phone and updating the database at the same time? There are also many surprises. I have encountered quite a few customers who had not visited a practice for many years, returned for checkups, and underwent expensive treatments.

Some technical matters are important in order for telemarketing to be effective. First, choose the right telemarketers. Telemarketing is a profession and not everyone can do it well – it's mostly appropriate for pensioners and students. Second, the scope of the position is usually three to four nights a week between the hours of 4 PM and 8 PM, so the maximum monthly salary will be 64 hours per month (less than a part-time position) and would not burden the practice financially.

In some cases, when the practice cannot recruit a designated telemarketer or when there is an interest in increasing the receptionist's or assistant's working hours, it is possible that they do the telemarketing work, but on the condition that this is not done during the practice's regular hours. This option is less recommended, but can prove successful in some cases.

4. **Cultivating the practice's recommenders** – As noted, customer retention is important, however it is worth clarifying that the retention of recommending customers is doubly important! Why? Because the contribution of customer recommendations to the practice's success is tremendous; customers who come to the practice through recommendations usually come prepared and begin treatment immediately. They bargain less compared to those who come through advertising, and more than that, the practice does not invest a cent in getting them to come in. It is no coincidence that every practice's dream is for its existing clients to recommend that their acquaintances receive care at the practice – and the more the better. The million-dollar question is, though, how to get the practice's clients to recommend it to their acquaintances.

Before answering this question, it is worth noting an important issue: customers are afraid of making a recommendation. Why? Because they fear that if their acquaintance is disappointed (for example, they receive bad treatment) this may be "their fault" and therefore, a customer will make a recommendation to his or her acquaintances only when he or she is 100% sure that their acquaintances will be happy with the treatment at the practice. Therefore, in order for customers to recommend the practice, the initial condition is to provide a level of service and treatment that is as high as possible for existing customers so that they will be sure to recommend the practice to their friends.

However, it does not end there. The most important part is to encourage and nurture those who have already recommended the practice.

What actually happens in these cases? Not much. Most practices ask customers from whom they heard about the practice, etc., but this is where it ends. The practice does nothing about the recommender, and thus begins the problem. To illustrate this let us take, for example, a theoretical case from another field. Let's say that six months ago you recommended that your acquaintance go to your car repair garage. From the moment, you made the recommendation you don't know whether your acquaintance went to the garage, whether he or she was satisfied, and so on. Quite by chance, another acquaintance asks you, "Do you know of a good garage?" What level of motivation and confidence would you feel in recommending that garage if you've heard nothing from the first friend? Probably not a high one and it is doubtful that you would recommend the same garage again.

Now imagine a situation where the same day that your acquaintance goes to the garage the owner calls you and says, "Hello Mr. Smith, how are you? You sent Mr. Brown to us. We appreciate it very much. By the way, he had a simple problem and the matter was fixed within two hours. Of course we gave him a special discount, and of course you'll get a discount the next time you visit."

This phone call will likely encourage you to recommend them again and not just for the discount, but mainly for the feeling that you did something good by making the recommendation, both for your acquaintance and for the garage.

So what's the problem in applying this to your dental practice starting tomorrow? Write down the names of the recommenders, call any recommender the same day their friends arrive at the practice or at the latest the following day, update them, and thank them for the recommendation. Write in their file that they made a recommendation and offer a certain discount on treatments, for example a dental hygiene treatment for 50% off. By the way, it doesn't matter whether the customer they recommended followed up with treatment or not; you should call and thank them in any case. If possible, and especially if the client has agreed to an extensive treatment plan, it is better that the dentist call as this will show gratitude and urge customers to continue recommending the practice.

5. **Membership or Loyalty Club** – Tens of percent of the total money spent in department stores is by members of their loyalty club. This means that that these stores, in fact, have no right to exist without club members. The principle behind the idea of a loyalty club is simple: be faithful to us and you will receive benefits in return.

This arrangement is good for both parties – the business earns repeated and loyal customers and the customers earn benefits and attractive prices on purchases. Instead of the business investing in recruiting new customers it will earn a bit less in favor of its existing customers. Customers, on their part, enjoy seeing a high price on the price tag and paying less upon displaying a member's card.

A members' club can also exist in a dental practice. Imagine each of your practice's clients holding a club card in their wallet: if customers know they have special privileges, will they go to receive treatment elsewhere? Probably not. By the way, public clinics operate a certain type of members' club. Take away their cards and free plaque removal, and you will see a significant drop in the number of visitors to these practices .The recommended benefits for club members vary from practice to practice. This depends on the type of practice, the type of treatments it offers, its size, etc. Benefits for practice members could be free consultation and checkups every six months, free emergency care, an 18% discount on a variety of practice treatments, or a 30% discount on dental hygienist treatments. Of course, when deciding on the practice's prices discounts for the practice's membership club should also be taken into account.

Another thing to remember is that the club can be a significant lever for recruiting new customers. It is easier to recruit new customers to a members' club than to a practice. Club benefits can be offered to places of work near the practice – who wouldn't like their dentist to be close to their workplace?

A practice that chooses to establish a membership club should formulate a series of benefits that are worthwhile, and not just give customers a fancy card. In addition, a considerable investment is required for the retention of club members: direct mail, e-mail, telemarketing, etc. Maintenance should be done on a consistent basis. Practices that don't build the members' club correctly and are not willing to invest in it should not start a club in the first place.

In conclusion, it can be said that customer retention laws are essentially similar to laws of maintaining a personal relationship: when either party (or both) takes the relationship for granted and stops investing in it, the connection breaks down. The same thing happens with clients: if you are passive, don't invest in communication, and don't appreciate the fact that they are your clients, it is reasonable to assume that the relationship will not last long. On the other hand, practices that succeed in keeping up constant, high-quality contact with their customers based on a win-win concept will receive regular visits from customers and their acquaintances, and as a result gain economic and business success.

Chapter 4

Positioning and Differentiation

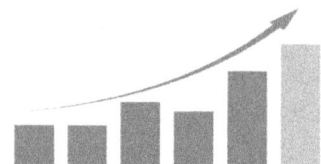

Positioning

The struggle is not between products but between perceptions. In simple terms and in connection to dental marketing, the competition has less to do with who the most professional dentist is, but which dentist is perceived as the most professional.

Have no doubt – perception is reality. Dentists may be extremely professional in terms of actions but if they cannot present a professional persona, the clients will perceive them as unprofessional and will not set foot in their practice. This equation works in the opposite direction as well – we all know of mediocre dentists who manage to create a professional image and turn their practice into a gold mine.

Perception is in fact an image. Let's take an example from the world of brands: Coca-Cola is considered the enemy of health but is a huge success nevertheless. This is because marketing experts have succeeded in creating a positive perception of the product as one that helps you enjoy life. On the other hand, other inexpensive sweetened drinks which are also considered to be bad for your health are perceived negatively by consumers because of their low prices and especially because they have never supported their image through advertising or other marketing activity.

The dentist is also located on the client's perceptual scale. He or she can be perceived as positive: professional, patient, sympathetic, and gentle – which will lead to success; or as negative: unprofessional, expensive, insensitive, rough, and impatient – which will keep customers away. From my experience with many dentists, one thing is clear: the most successful dentists are those who have succeeded in producing a positive perception of themselves.

The good news is that perception is something that can be generated. The first step in producing a positive attitude toward a dentist or practice is to internalize that it is crucial to success. Paradoxically, I have encountered quite a few professional dentists who fail in the creation of perception; they are so confident in their professional abilities that they do not feel they have to make an effort to be perceived as professional, and refrain from marketing themselves to customers.

However, precisely because clients cannot gage the dentist's professional qualities, the perception that he or she succeeds in creating is an exclusive reality for the client. It follows, then, that the concept is built on external characteristics. The clients assemble an image with fragments of information and generate a perception of the dentist and the practice.

For example, if the dentist is the director of the oral and maxillofacial department of a well-known hospital, the client will immediately conclude that he or she is a professional. Additional data, such as the fact that the dentist is a specialist or graduate of a prestigious dental school with more than 15 years of experience or has an innovative practice, may also improve his or her professional image in the customer's eyes. The trick is to know how to leverage this information and inform customers about it, in order to create an attractive image of the dentist and the practice. It is no accident that many professionals hang certificates of training on the walls of their offices – the goal is to improve their professional image in the customer's eyes.

Not surprisingly external features, which appear to be unimportant, contribute to perception. A customer entering a practice that is tastefully decorated, in which the staff is dressed in contemporary uniforms, and in which the dentist presents the diagnosis with an intra-oral camera on a plasma screen, will formulate a professional and innovative perception of the practice. Of course, the same logic works in the opposite direction.

There are three very simple ways for any practice to strengthen and improve its and the dentist's positioning in the customer's eyes.

1. **Promotional brochure** – You'll be surprised to hear this, but new customers entering the practice for the first time are very interested in who is going to examine and maybe treat them. Where did they get their training? How many years of experience do they have? How long has the practice existed? Does the practice perform dental implants and complete oral rehabilitation? And so on. In reality, however, a strange situation occurs – in the absolute majority of practices, customers enter an examination without all the information about the dentist or the practice. Often, they receive a proposal for a full rehabilitation program at a very high cost and are expected to make a decision on the spot.

    It is in the practice's interest, first and foremost, to inform new and existing customers about the practice's competitive advantages: what training the dentist received, how long the practice has existed, the variety of treatments performed at the practice, etc. All these important factors, which may strengthen the positioning and image of the practice, can be conveyed to the customer in a simple and clear manner with the help of an informative brochure.

    The brochure should not just be placed between the newspapers in the waiting room in the hopes that clients will take one on their own, but must be given prior to the examination together with the medical questionnaire: "Ms. Smith, you are invited to read about the practice before the examination." You can be sure that customers will read it and be very interested in the practice's background and in who might perform the treatment. Additionally, the brochure should be attached to the client's treatment plan, preferably within the folder, in order for them to receive supplementary information about the practice while they are receiving quotes from several practices and debating where to receive care.

    Imagine Mr. Smith receiving offers from three different practices. Two practices give him a simple treatment plan as most practices do, but your practice, in addition to the treatment plan, gives him a brochure in a folder, with supplementary information about the competitive advantages of the practice. Ladies and gentlemen, there is a high probability that the client will decide to turn to you for treatment, thanks to the professional impression that you have succeeded in formulating.

2. **Certificates** – It is no coincidence that training and education certificates can be found hanging on the walls of offices of accountants and lawyers. As stated, customers have no way of appreciating professionalism and one of the ways to help them do so is by hanging certificates that subconsciously convey the message, "I am educated and well-trained."

A considerable number of dentists see the presentation of training certificates as unnecessary and invest mainly in a beautiful and innovative practice. This thinking stems from two main reasons – the first is that the dentist examines the matter from a doctor's point of view ("You can receive a certificate after a two-day course") and not from the client's point of view ("Wow, a very educated dentist!"). The second reason is that most interior designers and architects who design practices do not consider the marketing aspect, only the aesthetic point of view.

There are many beautiful and innovative dental practices, but they neglect to emphasize professionalism. As stated, professionalism is the most important parameter for customers when choosing a dental practice. It is more important to new customers sitting in the waiting room to know that they arrived at a professional institution (documents hanging on the wall indicating that the dentist received training in dental implants at a well-regarded university, a diploma from a well-known dental school, or a license for general anesthesia) than to see beautiful paintings and an avant-garde statuette.

Of course, design is important as well and a practice should be beautiful and pleasing to the eye, but these features are not as important as training certificates. Allow for a combination of elements, but stick to the rule: certificates should be placed in strategic places such as the waiting room, treatment room, and office. In short, they should be placed where the customers are sitting. Beautiful, matching frames for these documents can contribute here as well.

3. **Uniforms** – Yes, even the dentist and practice staff have an impact on the practice's positioning and image. A dentist wearing an old and stained coat with an ink stain on the front pocket will be perceived in the clients subconscious as an old-fashioned and unprofessional dentist, therefore it is not worth economizing on uniforms – and although it's convenient to use disposable coats, they don't look good and do not broadcast professionalism.

Another important matter regarding uniforms: a dentist coat and jeans do not work together. A dentist dressed in jeans looks like someone who has been sitting in a cafe and when the time came, put on a coat and began to work. It is best to wear a full uniform, including dress pants. Doctors working in hospitals are obliged to wear full uniforms for a reason – not just for sterility.

Differentiation

Differentiation, as its name implies, makes all the difference, and is a necessary element for all dental practices. What is the difference between your dental practice and other dental practices? If your practice is similar to other practices and does not offer any unique features, then customers will focus on prices alone and simply choose the least expensive practice. On the other hand, if your practice is different and has more benefits than its competitors have, customers will turn to you for care and be willing to pay more. Hence, separating your practice from others may keep your clients from focusing on price.

To what is this similar? Imagine a situation in which consumers face two options for the purchase of a bottle of mineral water, where both are of similar size and taste. If the price of bottle A is $1 and the price of bottle B is $3, it is reasonable to assume that the consumer will buy the cheaper of the two: bottle A. After all, water is water (and as we said, in the absence of a unique feature customers focus on the price). Now, imagine that the consumers know that the more expensive bottle, B, contains unique features: it has essential vitamins, improves digestion, and comes from the top of Mount Everest. In this situation, it is likely that customers will choose bottle B even though its price is higher.

Your practice must also separate itself from the rest of the practices in order to attract a certain clientele for a particular type of treatment, and to keep customers away from the thought, "If there is no difference between the practices then I will choose the cheaper one," as much as possible. There are practices that do manage to differentiate themselves, such as children's dental practices and specialist practices, but the vast majority of dental practices appeal to everyone and offer a variety of treatments. The reason for this is understandable – dental practices are afraid to lose customers and therefore offer everything to everyone. They even boast, "All treatments under one roof"; but a known marketing rule is, "Everything is nothing." It is better to be an expert in one field than mediocre in a few areas.

According to consumer perception, and rightly so, a business that specializes in a specific field may offer a higher quality of care in that same field than a business that offers services in many different areas. Let's consider an example from different fields: when people want to buy shoes they prefer to go to a shoe store, or when interested in an electric appliance they prefer to go to a store specializing in electrical appliances. The same logic applies in additional scenarios – someone who wants to get a divorce will prefer to hire the services of a lawyer specializing in divorce rather than a general attorney.

The same applies to dentistry – a patient will prefer to undergo a dental implant procedure in a practice specializing in implantation and specifically one named "The Dental Implant Center," than in a dental practice that performs implants in addition to many other procedures. Parents will prefer to take their children to a practice specializing in children's care, than to a regular practice that also provides dental treatments for children. True, the very act of differentiation creates a concession of certain market segments, but on the other hand, differentiation attracts more customers looking for the specific service that is provided and the practice can charge a higher premium for its expertise.

Business reality shows that specialized businesses are far more profitable than those trying to sell a wide range of products to all customers. In the automotive industry, for example, companies such as **Lamborghini** or **Porsche** are considered more profitable than **Ford**, **Renault**, or **Peugeot**, which produce a wide range of products and services. The reason for this stems from the fact that distinct businesses understand the unique needs of their customers and provide them with more quality services and products, so customers are willing to pay higher prices for services that are more professional. Additionally, the expenses of specialized businesses are significantly lower than those who offer a wide range of services and products to the public.

The decision to differentiate the dental practice is a complex one and which depends on many factors such as characteristics of competitors in the region, the practice's strengths and weaknesses, characteristics of the target audience, etc., but in any event, differentiation must take place. There are many options for differentiation; you just need to decide which option to focus on.

I know of a number of dental practices that have learned to do so. A certain practice I've encountered distinguishes itself as one that only hires graduates of a certain prestigious university. Another practice distinguishes itself with a design inspired by a fancy cafe – customers are offered treatment plans while they sit at the reception desk on bar stools and drink coffee. There are, of course, dental practices that differentiate themselves by the type of treatments they provide, including: specialist surgery, children's care, root canal treatments, orthodontics, gum care, and so on.

However, almost all dental practices are unable to resist the temptation to offer additional services. I once encountered a successful dental practice run by a children's specialist who insisted on introducing root canal treatments. This created an identity crisis for the practice: half of it was a pediatric practice and the other, a specialist's practice. The children who came to the practice did not feel comfortable with the other half of the practice, and the adults who came for root canal treatments were uncomfortable with the colorful design and children running around.

PART TWO

BUSINESS POLICY AND MANAGEMENT OF PRACTICE STAFF

Chapter 5

Receptionist Conduct

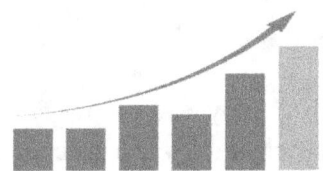

Let's start from the end: With all due respect to the medical staff, the receptionist is the most important person in the practice, at least from a business perspective. This position is actually the motor driving the practice's wheels – if the wheels creak and move slowly, the whole practice falters. The receptionist's position contains important and influential aspects effecting the practice's function and success. It is no accident that behind every successful practice is an efficient and effective receptionist, and of course the other way around.

However, working at the reception desk is also the most difficult and complex job at the practice. Workers at the receptionist's desk are supposed to function like Wonder Woman – they need to simultaneously deal with confirmations, manage appointments, answer the phone, close treatment plans, maintain contact with the laboratory, collect payments, handle the practice's managers requests, marketing, and so on.

An owner of a certain practice who hired my services in the past defined the receptionist's position in the following way, which I find to be interesting and true: "There will always be holes in the 'net' of the receptionist's work; the question is what size the holes are and how many fish slip away. As long as this happens on a reasonable level, the practice will function well and be profitable." This is an important statement; because of the complexity of the position, things always fall between the cracks – the question is, how many things? The trick is to minimize the damage.

In order to minimize loss and of course increase the practice's sales cycle, the receptionist's job must be performed correctly, effectively, and not according to "the way things have always been done," as unfortunately happens in quite a few practices. I will address several aspects of the receptionist's work that have a significant impact on the practice's business performance.

Role Definition

Imagine a situation in which three employees are in charge of 30 different tasks. They can choose from two strategies: The first, the three of them will storm the 30 tasks and perform them together.

The second option is for each employee to receive ten tasks and perform only them. The second option, in which each employee has her or his own tasks, is undoubtedly preferable. There are several reasons for this: First, when everyone does everything, the chances that things will fall between the cracks rises. Second, if someone is skilled in a particular field and weak in another, it is best to focus on what they are good at and leave the tasks in which they are weak to someone who excels at them. Third, if there is failure or success in a particular area, it is easier to know whom to contact and how it could be repaired or improved.

In most practices, the reception desk adopts a strategy of receptionists that cover all areas. All the receptionists preform confirmations, they all deal with insurance, and all of them follow up with customers who have not closed treatment plans. There is nothing worse than this.

The more positions are differentiated and the more responsibilities are divided between receptionists, the better off the employees will be, leading to the practice functioning well in general. Obviously, there are tasks that all receptionists must perform such as answering the phones and setting up appointments, but there are additional areas that must be divided up based on the employees' qualifications. If Ruthie "blows through" paperwork, it is best that she alone handles insurance. Moreover, if customers seem to prefer speaking to Anne on the phone, she should perform RE-CALLS to customers who have not closed treatment plans.

The division of responsibilities is even more significant when it comes to medium-sized or large practices (three units or more). In such a situation, you should even physically separate your employees from the rest of the practice, and divide the work according to dentists and the types of treatments. Receptionists Ruthie and Anne handle the insurance for customers who undergo preservative treatments with Dr.

Hay and Dr. Jones, and receptionists Margret and Bob will take care of customers who undergo implantations and rehabilitation with Dr. Isabella and Dr. Essad.

It is also recommended that once a week the person in charge of each area (collection, insurance, implants, rehabilitation) meet with the practice's owner for half an hour and present them with data and problems such as the number of treatment plans that were closed that week, customers who are still thinking about the plan proposal they received (John wants to pay cash and is asking for another discount; Silvia is debating between plan A and B), payments that have yet to be collected, and so on.

Phone Response

This may sound strange, but the telephone – yes, that little device – is in charge of the dental practice's success or, heaven forbid, its failure. Think about it – everything beings there: appointments, new customer inquiries, confirmations, contact with the lab, suppliers, etc. No one comes in for treatment impulsively; it always begins on the phone. Since everything starts there, it is the primary channel that drives the whole business and therefore the utmost importance should be attributed to it. In addition, the phone is the practice's front line, where initial contact with new customers takes place and where they begin to formulate either a negative or a positive first impression of the practice.

It is important to clarify that any missed phone calls can have enormous economic implications for the practice. In a trivial case, when a customer calls interested in a full-blown rehabilitation and is not treated correctly, that phone call can cost the practice a significant amount of money and significantly affect that month's bottom line. The same principle also works in reverse. No practice has the luxury of failing to answer the phone. Paradoxically, phone response is the weak point of a majority of dental practices.

Here are a few points to pay attention to in the context of the practice's conduct, in order to minimize missed phone calls:

Telephone response format

The manner of phone response must be respectful, presentable, and in a consistent format; for example, "Dr. Jones's Practice, Anne speaking."

This is because a phone response must include two pieces of information: first, the name of the business the customer has called, and second, with whom they are speaking. Why is this important? First, the customers want to know whether they have indeed reached the business they dialed (Dr. Jones's dental practice), and second, they want to know that a staff member is on the line. A client cannot create an emotional connection with the practice, but can make a connection with "Anne." It is no coincidence that clients ask, "Wait a minute, who am I speaking with?" It's much more comfortable to know whom you are speaking to and the conversation becomes more personal when you know the name of the person on the other end of the line.

However, phone response in most practices is short and limp. I've even heard some receptionists answering with, "Hello." It is worth noting that companies in various countries have significantly improved their phone response in recent years, and that customers are exposed to this type of response regularly. Therefore, dental practices cannot remain behind in this regard, especially when it comes to an opportunity – which is quite simple to implement – to help the practice's image.

Considering this, no concessions should be made on this matter. So what should we do? A small sign should be put up at the receptionist station with the desirable phrase for answering the phone, and you should make sure that the receptionists begin to answer respectfully and in a presentable manner. If the receptionists answer the phone in this way for a whole month, they will absorb the new style and it will come naturally to them.

Quality of Phone Response

Another important issue is the quality of phone response; in other words, what are the answers given to customers' questions on the phone? How do receptionists deal with customers? For example, what are the answers that your receptionists give customers who call and ask questions such as, "How much does an implant cost?" or, "Do you take insurance?"

An easy way to know what your customers are going through is simply to make undercover phone calls. Ask someone to call the practice and pose questions to the receptionists. Ask them to tell you how long it took the receptionists to answer (if at all), if they were pleasant and tolerant, if they answered all their questions, and so on. If there is something wrong, you might want to remind the staff of the phone procedures and the message package associated with the practice.

For example, discuss how to convey that there are specialists working at the practice and why this is an advantage, or what to tell customers who ask whether the practice takes insurance. Do you inform customers of prices over the phone? And so on.

Missed Phone Calls

The issue of missed phone calls is considered the most painful problem for dental practices. As mentioned, a missed call could mean an expensive treatment plan not being performed at the practice and affecting the bottom line of the sales cycle for the month. How do you miss a phone call? Very easily. Note that most dental practices make do with an answering machine when the practice is closed or when the line is busy. But studies show that 80% of customers do not leave messages when they encounter an answering machine, so in fact you only hear from the 20% of callers who did leave a message.

What happens to the other 80% of customers who tried to reach you?

Think about it: what happens when a new customer calls the practice to schedule an appointment, however the first time the line is busy, the second time it is busy too, and the third time the answering machine picks up? I'll tell you: he'll think, "Wait a minute, what if I join this practice, and need emergency treatment, or a crown gets loose? I won't be able to reach them! I should keep looking."

So what should we do about this? The solution is simple: there are many companies who provide a message service when the practice is closed or when the line is busy. The practice receives a message (email, SMS, or fax) about who called and can then get back to them, preventing a situation in which clients repeatedly try to reach the practice and fail.

Organizational Structure

A practice should strive to work as an optimal workforce – one that does not employ redundant workers and spend unnecessary salaries on the one hand, but doesn't have a shortage of labor that causes things to fall between the cracks or the loss of business, on the other hand. In most cases, there is a direct correlation between the volume of sales turnover and the number of employees required at the practice. A large sales turnover means more customers, more treatments, more phone calls, more administration, and therefore more workers needed, and of course, the opposite is true as well.

There are three main types of organizational structures in dental practices:

1. **Dentist + assistant** – The basic and primary structure of a dental practice is one dentist and one assistant who also acts as a receptionist. In practices of this kind, the assistant arrives at the practice even when it is closed, and takes care of matters such as RE-CALLS, insurance, etc. Incidentally, in this situation, the assistant answers the phone even during treatments, and this is not an optimal situation. Despite this, in low cycle situations there are not many phones call and there is no economic justification for employing an additional receptionist.

2. **Dentist + assistant + receptionist** – In practices with a higher level of activity it is recommended to add a receptionist to the practice. This activity creates a high number of phones calls and a lot of administrative work. The practice requires a dedicated worker to handle administrative matters. In many cases, the receptionist will be responsible for the closing of treatment plans and following up on treatment programs that have not been closed.

3. **Dentist + assistant + receptionist + practice manager** – This is applicable to a mid-size-plus practice, with a high sales turnover. Apart from the need for administrative growth, such high sales cycles require staff management, shift management, supervision, overseeing RE-CALL work, managing a newsletter, collection, etc. These are things the dentist will not have time to do. Additionally, in most cases practice managers will have better sales skills than the receptionists will, so they will be responsible for closing the practice's treatment plans.

Beyond the three main organizational structures, there are several other structures as well: in large practices with a high sales turnover and an administrative workload, two receptionists work during every shift alongside a full-time manager. Another thing that is needed in big practices that have a large amount of new appointments is a sales manager. The sales manager will only deal with the sale of treatment plans and follow up on programs that have not been closed. This role is very important because a practice that has a large amount of checkups leads to a large amount of customers who are going to be uncertain about treatment, therefore a full-time employee is required to monitor these customers closely. From experience, if this role is staffed by the right sales person this can make the difference between a mediocre and a successful dental practice.

A note in conclusion: In determining the correct organizational structure for the practice there is no one answer but rather it is a matter of perception. There are practice owners who think that one receptionist is sufficient for a certain load of customers, and owners of other practices will consider two receptionists appropriate for the same workload. According to my approach, it is better to have an extra employee than not enough. Why? Because if there are superfluous employees, the worst-case scenario is that that the practice loses a monthly wage, which only happens if a worker really does not do anything. However, if there is a shortage of workers, the practice will miss phone calls, have clients who do not receive good service, and will end up with no follow-up for treatment programs that have not been closed properly, etc. Eventually the practice is liable to lose a few treatment plans a month that could amount to significant financial impact.

Of course, there is no need to hold on to extra employees, but rather to manage the entire staff effectively and to ensure that there is no hidden – and certainly not overt – unemployment. Additionally, you shouldn't overload the practice staff. A team that works under pressure is quickly worn out and cannot provide effective and patient service, as well as generate quality sales calls. Unfortunately, the most common situation is that dental practices have fewer staff than needed, which creates pressure and overloads the receptionist's position, causing many issues to go unmanaged and ultimately the sales and profitability cycles of the practice are affected.

Disclosing Prices over the Phone

Many receptionists do not disclose prices to customers over the phone because "this is not a marketplace." However, customers think differently: the vast majority of customers who encounter a refusal following this legitimate request will ultimately not choose to be treated at the practice. It is redundant to note that failure to reach customers means a significant financial loss to the practice.

On the other hand, it is difficult to say how much an implant will cost, because there are different kinds of implants, and the customer may need a bone transplant, etc. Therefore, the receptionist should use a middle ground – on the one hand answer the customer's questions and encourage them to come for a checkup, but on the other hand not commit to a specific price. The recommended wording is: *"Mr. Smith, implants costs between X and Y dollars, depending on the type of implant and the complexity of the treatment. I'd be happy to set up an appointment with Dr. Jones, who has 17 years of experience in dental implants. By the way, you may not need an implant at all."*

In such a situation, the clients receive what they want and the practice is not perceived as unreliable for trying to hide its prices. No less important is that the customer feels obligated to arrive and see if perhaps they do not need an implant after all. The receptionist can always add, *"Mr. Smith, you are heading towards a complex and expensive process; I suggest you get a second professional opinion. When can you come in for a checkup – in the morning or in the evening?"*

Free Checkups

In my experience, dental practices that choose to perform paid checkups do so for two reasons, the first reason being, "The dentist's time is precious" and the second is, "A customer who is not prepared to pay for a checkup is not a customer whom we should be interested in." The first reason is perhaps justified; the second reason is not accurate at all. But it really does not matter – the collection policy for checkups should be considered according to clean economic calculations.

Let's conduct a simple calculation: if ten people call and want to come in for a consultation and hear that the cost is, say, $200, in a best-case scenario only four of them, on average, will indeed set a date for the examination. So out of ten callers the practice adds $800 to its income, but on the other hand, prevents six new potential customers from coming in.

The question is, how much money could the practice have made from those six customers who did not show up? In a simple calculation: if only one of them signed up for a treatment plan, the profit would be much higher than $800.

Instead of trying to educate customers the practice should adjust its policy to the rules of the game and consumer behavior. The practice's main interest is that as many customers as possible enter it and familiarize themselves with the services it offers. It's all about statistics – more customers entering the practice result in more closed treatment plans.

By the way, the question here is not whether customers are justified in their demand to not pay for the examination (they aren't), and not even whether dentists are right to demand payment for their time (they are). The question is, what actually happens? And you should act only based on this; if the payment for the checkup prevents customers from getting examined, then it is worthwhile to be smart rather than right, and remove this barrier preventing clients from coming to the practice.

So why, you may ask, do customers pay for testing and consultation in other medical fields? The answer is that the rules of the game in other industries are different from those of the dental industry. The level of competition in the field of Gynecology, for example, is very low compared to that of Dentistry, and the level of competition in a particular sector has the greatest impact on the ability to collect payment for an initial examination. Needless to say, the level of competition in the dental industry is the highest among the various branches of medicine and therefore not coincidentally, more than 95% dental practices do not charge for the initial exam.

Additionally, the "offset" method, where the payment for the first appointment is added to the treatment cost if the client decides to receive care at the practice, is not very effective. A client once told me, "It's a matter of principle – I know I need treatment at the cost of thousands of dollars or more and I am examining options for treatment with three practices. Why should I pay each practice for the initial exam? The practice which impresses me the most is where I will receive treatment and pay the full price."

However, there are unique practices (run by department managers, specialists, etc.) that charge high prices for tests and where customers agree to pay, so if customers are willing to pay then by all means, don't turn them down.

Appointment Management

One of the most acute issues, when it comes to the conduct of the receptionist's position, is appointment management. The potential that things will go wrong and customers will not end up in the dentist's chair is great, so it is worthwhile to work thoroughly and systematically to ensure that appointment management is run efficiently. The following are five guiding principles for effective management of appointments.

1. Handling No-Shows

The receptionist calls Ms. Smith to remind her of the appointment which is supposed to take place the next day. As in many cases, Ms. Smith informs the receptionist that she will not be able to make it. What should be done in a case such? The receptionist wishes to set up a new appointment for Ms. Smith. But what happens when Ms. Smith cannot set up a new appointment because she is in the middle of jogging? She tells the receptionist that she'll call back, and as far as the receptionist is concerned, that is the end of that.

Oops, this is exactly where things begin to fall apart. The receptionist passed the ball into Ms. Smith's court, and worse, in terms of the practice, after her appointment was canceled, Ms. Smith is expected to call and set up a new appointment herself. As you can probably guess, in many cases Ms. Smith will not call for a new appointment – she has more important (and enjoyable) things to do. This leads to a missed client for the practice.

Due to cases such as this one, the number one rule in managing appointments is to never pass the ball into the client's court. The control must always stay in the receptionist's hands. Anyone who has not arrived on time must be registered in a separate list and closely monitored until a new appointment is made for them: "You're not in front of a calendar, Ms. Smith? No problem, I'll call you tomorrow morning and set up new appointment." Ms. Smith's name should be removed from the list only after a new appointment has been scheduled for her.

2. X-rays and scans

Another scenario that could cause customers to disappear from some practices is when they are sent for an x-ray or a scan (CT or panoramic). The customers receive brief instructions: "Please go for an x-ray/scan and call to schedule an appointment."

In this case as well, the ball moves over to the customer and they may never call. Instead, the receptionist should tell the customer, "Go for an x-ray/scan and I'll schedule an appointment for you in another week or two. Please bring the results with you then."

This way the receptionist achieves two things: First, the customers are not lost to the practice, since they have an appointment. Second, the practice encourages the customer to go for the x-ray or scan as soon as possible rather than delay it, increasing the chances that the appointment will be kept in the near future. How many customers do you know that were sent for an x-ray or scan and have not done so yet? Yes, I know of a lot, too.

3. Scheduling Appointments

If there is a schedule considered negative and unprofitable for the practice, it is one filled with half-hour appointments. Such a schedule causes many problems, especially for the profitability of the practice. When many customers are scheduled for the same day it is likely that some will not arrive, which could disrupt the entire work schedule. Additionally, studies have found that receiving and discharging a customer ("Hi and bye") takes about six minutes on average – so for every ten patients an hour is wasted!

Therefore, a practice should strive for a state of "assembled appointments" when medically possible, and after the client gives their consent, it is worthwhile to set up long appointments, an hour or two long, and perform several treatments simultaneously. For example, "Mr. Smith, what do you prefer, coming here eight times for half an hour, or instead two two-hour sessions? Don't worry; we'll take breaks as needed." In most cases, customers will respond positively to the offer.

In this way, the practice can increase productivity considerably, and clients will be happy that they do not have to come to the practice eight times for a simple filling. In addition, this is a good opportunity to make an appointment for customers during the morning hours which are relatively dead hours in most practices and thus clear the schedule for the popular "golden hours" in the evening). By the way, the chances of a customer canceling a two-hour appointment are significantly lower than the chance of a cancelation of a half-hour appointment. In most cases, they will take time off from work to undergo a treatment on the day of the longer appointment.

4. Reminders

No system has been found yet to bring all patients in for testing or treatments. The reason for this is simple: statistically speaking, there will always be those who will not be able to come to their appointments for reasons such as family emergencies, urgent meetings, etc. However, if the number of customers who do not show up to their appointments exceeds 10%, it is worth checking out the reminder system being used by the receptionist.

Studies on consumer behavior show that a commitment from clients puts them in a state of discomfort and motivates them to act. Therefore, it is worth adding the following sentence at the end of the reminder call: "Dr. Jones will be waiting for you at X, please do not be late. You are coming right?" Once the customer's answer is "Yes," it creates a kind of commitment on their part to make it to the appointment.

5. Delays

During my work with dentists, I have discovered an amazing statistic: there are practices where the amount of delays is intolerable and disrupts the practice's work, and there are practices where clients are hardly ever late. Why does this happen? Who is to blame for delaying customers? If you ask the practice staff, they will say the customers are guilty, of course. However, as the saying goes, the camel does not see its hump.

The truth is a bit painful; practices are the main culprits in most clients' delays. A practice that does not respect the client's time will not win the client's respect for its time. In an observation I performed at a practice that suffered from a severe delay problem, I heard a customer say, "My next appointment is Tuesday at 4:30 so I'll come in around five o'clock. Appointments never begin on time here."

People don't arrive late to a movie because they know the movie will start on time. On the other hand, they will arrive late at a practice where they know their appointment will not begin on time anyway. It is therefore important that the practice first makes sure that the client's appointment takes place at the appointed time, and only then can the clients be asked to be punctual. Except for cases of dentists who are chronically late for work, the main reason for delays is that practices do not manage their schedule correctly and overload appointments without taking into account facts that are known in advance: there will always be unforeseen emergency cases, appointments running longer than planned, and so on.

Therefore, the recommended strategy is to care well for 20 patients rather than provide poor care for 24. Accordingly, each workday should have two windows of 20-30 minutes each, so that all delays and emergency cases drain into these two windows and not create pressure and disorder.

In addition, customers must be informed of any delays along with an apology. In today's hectic world, a client who makes an appointment also makes a plan to pick up his wife for shopping or to pick up his kids from school. It is not surprising that people in the waiting room look nervous and impatient when there are delays, and rightly so. Needless to say, a delay can ruin the positive image and professionalism you have succeeded in producing at the customer's expense, and even cause the customer to move to a different practice. Additionally, a customer disappointed by the practice's disregard for their valuable time will be less willing to pay a high price for the treatments offered to them.

However, when an appointment is delayed it is possible (and worthwhile) to soften the blow. In fact, the customer understands that there can be delays, but they will only show understanding when they are informed of a delay in advance. The receptionist's role is to know when Mr. Smith is supposed to enter and whether there may be a delay. If a delay is expected, the receptionist should notify the customer at least 15 minutes before the appointment: "I apologize, Mr. Smith, but your appointment will be delayed by 15 minutes due to an emergency appointment."

A practice that does not soften the blow and does not apologize in advance sends their clients the message that their time is not important to it. These customers will not be willing to accept the delay. But what about the customer's lateness? First, although you waited for them in vain, try not to show that you are upset; it is not your job to educate them and they do not owe you anything. Secondly, do not delay a customer who arrives on time because of another customer who was late. The tardy clients can understand why they are delayed, and this may even teach them not to do so again, but a client who arrived on time should not be punished because of someone else's lateness. It is very unfair to delay them. In addition, chronically late customers should be scheduled for the end of the day.

Managing an Effective Collection System

Collection problems are the worst thing that can happen to a dental practice and in many cases may even lead to its collapse. The good news is that collection management based on my "sensitivity and determination" strategy may reduce the problem to a minimum.

A practice that does not collect payment correctly loses twice: it does not gain the money owed to it, and even worse, it loses money spent on lab expenses, wages, etc., on the customers who have not paid for treatments. As if this is not enough, it also loses the client – a client who owes money will not return to the practice.

My experience with collection problems shows that as far as the practice's staff is concerned (primarily the dentist), when they are "buddies" with the customers, the collection problems are worse.

Cellular service providers have no collection problems – they collect payment by standing order and disconnect the device if debt is not paid. This is what happens with the water company, the municipality, etc. Retail chains also have no collection problems: it is impossible to enter a supermarket, pick up some items, and not pay for them at the checkout counter. Customers are not embittered about this – they understand that that's how it works.

The problems start when you give customers a loophole and thereby put them in a trap. They want to pay and even open a savings plan to fund the treatment, but delay the payment to the practice since it allows them to do so, and use the money for other purposes; when the bill grows (especially on reconstruction work) they do not have the money available and cannot pay. Once again, the practice has lost twice: it did not receive the money and lost the client as well.

Since I have encountered quite a few collection problems in my business consultations at dental practices, I have developed a collection policy of "Sensitivity and Determination," which, if implemented without shortcuts, will assure that your dental practice's collection problems will disappear.

The collection policy is based on six main principles:

1. **Pre-payment** – The ultimate goal is to charge in advance for each treatment plan. Imagine how easy and comfortable life will be, both for you and for your customer, if the customer arranges a prepayment. When the client does not regulate the prepayment, this must be dealt with at almost every encounter: "Mr. Smith, you have to pay for the treatment." "Wait a minute, but I paid already, didn't I? How much do I owe? Oops, I don't have my checkbook with me." And so on.

   Therefore, the best solution is to arrange advance payment. When Mr. Smith says, "I want to pay according to the progress of the treatments," you should answer, "No problem, Mr. Smith; you aren't paying for the whole treatment now, only arranging the payment. The treatment will take about eight months. I will be happy to arrange 12 payments so that you are finished with the treatment before you are done paying." It is always a good idea to add this to the argument: "We deal with the payments once, now, and then focus solely on the medical treatment."

2. **High initial payment** – Customers who decide to carry out a treatment plan at the cost of a few thousand dollars or more usually do not have this amount in their checking account. The initial payment should be high in order to improve the practice's cash flow as well as to ensure payment. The demand for a down payment can always be justified as high lab costs, payment for the surgical work at the beginning of treatment, or as a condition for a special discount for the customer: "No problem, Mr. Smith, I'll give you another discount; if you pay 50% in cash I'll be able to arrange five payments for you." Incidentally, the policy of advance payment upon signing for the transaction is also practiced in other areas, for example the purchase of a model apartment.

   Additionally, it's a good idea to exercise discretion with respect to payments and payment methods – it is recommended to prefer credit cards to checks, and avoid many high payments with checks. A practice that offers the customer a payment option with 18 checks should not be surprised if some of the later ones bounce.

3. **Do not proceed with the treatment before a payment has been made** – You should by no means proceed with the treatment if the customer has not arranged payment for it, especially when the treatment is accompanied by lab work (which

you will have to pay for). Just to be clear, collection for the treatment should take place only before the treatment and not afterwards: "Mr. Smith, we have to settle the financial issue before transferring the data to the lab and ordering materials for the rehabilitation."

4. **Advance notice** – While making the reminder call, go through the personal file and check if the customer owes money. If so, the receptionist should say, "Mr. Smith, please bring a form of payment with you to arrange payment for your treatment." This will ensure that Mr. Smith will not arrive and say he has no checks or credit cards with him.

5. **Supervision** – Every two or three weeks, the practice owner should go over the collection situation with the person responsible for it in the practice: who owes the practice money, how much, and why. Those who wake up every few months and discover to their surprise that they are owed a significant amount of money should not be surprised that collection is difficult – the longer it takes, the more difficult it is to collect the payment owed. Therefore, the aim is to perform the collection as close to the time of treatment as possible.

6. **Disengagement** – "The customer is always right" and the practice staff should always be accommodating and do everything to satisfy them. However, this is not a one-sided relationship – the clients also have a commitment to the practice: they must pay for the treatments. A client who does not fulfill his or her part in the agreement should not to be a client at the practice.
Customers, with whom all collection attempts have failed and still insist on not paying, should be cut off before they become the reason for lost debt.

How to Transfer Clients Correctly

One of the most troubling issues for dentists is the difficulty in transferring patients to other dentists. On the one hand, it is flattering that the patients only want you, but on the other hand, if you want to move forward, expand the practice, and maximize profitability per hour of work, you cannot continue to perform fillings and root canals forever.

The problem is very well known and widespread: dentists with extensive experience, surgical wizards, and full oral rehabilitation specialists who have managed to build a successful practice with a number of younger and more energetic dentists still find themselves with a calendar full of small, unprofitable treatments. Sometimes I encounter dentists who perform treatments intended for dental hygienists. Why? Because patients, who have been accustomed to them from the start, are not willing to be treated by another.

Not that I have anything against preventative dental treatments (fillings, root canals, etc.), but it is better for every practice that the division of labor be both medical and business-oriented. The veteran dentist should deal with complex dental procedures that require more experience and skill such as surgery and major rehabilitation, while the younger dentists should deal with the simpler treatments.

What should be done, then? How do we manage to transfer patients, whom we have been treating for years, to another dentist? Well, before I get to the tactics of what to do and how, it's worth clarifying one thing: in most cases customers do not agree to transfer because the dentist does not completely want to transfer them. How do I know? Many veteran dentists simply do not conduct root canals or serious surgery but transfer this work to another dentist, and all of their customers are willing to transfer to other dentists. I have not encountered a dentist, who has not performed root canal treatments in years, performing one because a client insisted that only they perform it.

So how is it that the patient transfers to another dentist in these cases and does not agree to transfer when individual fillings or crowns are necessary? The answer is clear; the dentist does not really want to transfer the client. Therefore, before starting the transfer process, both the dentist and the practice staff must make a clear and unequivocal decision: Dr. Jones does not perform fillings, individual crowns, and certainly not plaque removal – period! You should clearly define which treatments the dentist no longer performs.

Now let us discuss how the patient should be transferred. The biggest mistake practices make is the way in which they explain to the patients why they should undergo a treatment with another dentist. The client says, "Who is Dr. Hay? I do not know him/her. I want Dr. Jones to treat me!" And what is the most common answer they receive from the receptionist or assistant? "Dr. Jones no longer performs fillings." Or, "The appointment book is full," and so on.

Is there any wonder that the clients don't want to be transferred over to Dr. Hay? Their interpretation is simple: *The dentist is already so successful that he no longer cares about me*, and, *The practice is considering the good of the dentist and not my own*. To this is added the patient's frustration: *I've been here for twenty years with my whole family, I've referred many acquaintances to the practice, and this is what I deserve? Does the dentist not have time for me?* No wonder this creates anger in the patient who threatens to leave the practice if Dr. Jones will not treat him. From there it's not long before the dentist caves and says, "Oh well, I really don't want to lose him and his whole family. Set up appointment for fillings and small treatments for him (and his whole family)."

None of this would have happened if the practice staff had handled the incident differently and changed their attitude toward the client. First, at the time of scheduling the office staff should not conduct discussions and consultations with the patients about who will perform treatment. "Mr. Smith, you will start with a cleaning with Linda the hygienist, the next appointment will be with Dr. Hay to do the work on the three fillings and the root canal, then Dr. Jones will perform the surgical stage, etc." Simply state the facts when speaking with the customer.

Moreover, here comes the greatest difference: when the client asks who Dr. Hay is and says he wants to be treated only by Dr. Jones, the approach to his request must be completely different. Notice the next important nuance: the practice staff should convey the message that they will be treated by Dr. Hay not because Dr. Jones is too busy for them, but because the division of work is such that every dentist does the things they are best at in order to benefit the patient. When the clients understand that their transfer to another dentist is performed for their personal benefit and not for the benefit of the dentist or the practice, this will go over relatively easily. You, of course, have to support the new dentist and give the patient a good reason or two for this move.

It goes like this: "Mr. Smith, we want you to receive the best treatment and Dr. Hay will perform the fillings because that's what he specializes in here at the practice and does best. He uses the latest methods and, by the way, he is also a student coach at a renowned dental school. Believe me, if I need a filling I go to him as well. When you get to the implantation and rehabilitation stage, Dr. Jones will take care of you. Of course, Dr. Jones is involved in all the stages of the treatment you are undergoing here at the practice." An option for further enhancing the professional perception of the dentist to whom the patients is transferred is to prepare a profile page – a type of resume – that will be given to patients and emphasize the dentist's professionalism and make it clear to the patient that they are in good hands.

Once patients realize that they will receive better care with the other dentist (yes, sometimes you have to set your ego aside), they will not hesitate for a moment about transferring, and even thank you for your honesty and concern for them. Finally, there may be a few tactics that will not work for some patients (for example, patients suffering from phobias) which you can give up on, but if you stick to the above approach the vast majority of patients can be transferred, clearing time for more significant and profitable treatments at the practice.

Internal Marketing

The practice staff has a huge impact on the customer's decision about where to receive treatment and what treatment to undergo. Clients tend to consult with the practice staff (receptionists, assistants, practice administrators, and dental hygienist) more than with the dentist. The reason for this is that customers maintain a kind of distance from the dentist and feel more comfortable consulting with the staff: "I'm worried about the sinus elevation. What is does it include? In all honesty, is he a good dentist? Does he have any experience with this procedure?"

Of course, in most cases, the practice staff has a positive opinion of the dentist and the practice, and they will recommend the practice. The question is in what manner is this done and how positive is the recommendation? When someone recommends something, the conviction of the recommendation is just as crucial as the messages conveyed. For example, in a case where a client asks the assistant whether the dentist is a good surgeon, one assistant will answer in a lukewarm, tentative manner, "Look, you have nothing to worry about; he's a good dentist. I do not know him enough because he comes to us once a month, but I have not heard of any problems with him. In short, you have nothing to be afraid of."

Another assistant in another practice will answer in a much more determined manner, "Are you asking about our surgeon Dr. Jones? My dear, he is one of the best surgeons in the country! He is a senior practitioner in the hospital and is a mouth and jaw specialist. He has been a surgeon for over 15 years and has done so many sinus lifts that it's like child's play for him. By the way, he even lectures to dentists overseas on dental implants and sinus lifts. I've been here for several years now, and judging by the amount of chocolate that customers bring him after treatment, you can set your mind at ease."

It is quite clear which recommendation will cause the client to decide immediately to undergo the sinus lift at the practice, and which recommendation will cause the client to hesitate and perhaps want to get another opinion from another practice.

If this is the case, the practice must not leave its fate in the hands of the staff and hope that they are able to convey clear messages to customers. The practice owner must guide the staff and make sure that they have enough information to pass on to customers if necessary. The first thing the practice owner needs and must do is create team spirit.

Your goal is to create a team spirit that is so high that your team will believe with all their hearts that the treatments performed at your practice are the best treatments at the best prices. Even if your prices are higher than your direct competitors, your team must understand and believe that treatment in the practice is worth every penny and that the customers, in fact, pay less than they should compared to what they get. If your team thinks the customers pay an exorbitant price, naturally their recommendations to customers will be lukewarm.

So how do you create team spirit? Very simple: a customer comes for front bridge work and the result is amazing? Great – stop all activity at the practice and ask the whole staff to come and see the beautiful work. More than that, show them the "before" pictures and point out the difference.

Ladies and gentlemen, this is not a matter of arrogance. It's a simple issue: the practice is selling dental treatments, and the result is the final product. Your staff must see and understand what customers end up with. Only if your team sees the deliverables will they be able to recommend the dentists and treatments to the practice's clients in a convincing and unequivocal manner. If not, they will only continue defending why the treatments are more expensive than in other practices and why there are delays with the appointments.

There are other situations you should share with your entire team in order to create team spirit. These situations are less pleasant, but necessary: Did a customer come to the practice after receiving bad dental care at another practice? For example, is an implant in a strange place? Call the whole team in and show them the case. Do not tell the team who the dentist is, so as not to make it personal – in general, you should be careful about competitors – but it is important that the staff know that the quality of dental treatment performed at your practice is not to be taken for granted and that a client who decides not to receive care at your practice risks receiving bad dental care.

In conclusion, the team that will best market the practice is one who believes that the treatments at your practice are the best and that the treatments in other practices are not as good.

Additionally, information should be provided to the practice staff so that they can transmit accurate and appropriate messages to customers. It may be difficult to believe, but I have encountered quite a few receptionists in dental practices who do not know the exact difference between a specialist and a general dentist, or what the prices of the competitors are, or what the difference is between a zirconia crown and a regular porcelain crown except for the price. How can your team face a customer and recommend the surgeon at the practice, making it clear that the prices are perfectly reasonable, and that zirconia crowns should be chosen for the front teeth, if they do not have the accurate information?

There are practices that take this matter a few steps further and actually hold a class for the staff once a month. They gather during the lunch break for about an hour and present interesting cases and medical treatments that took place at the practice, excellent results of treatments, etc. Of course, this is the optimal thing to do, but a practice that does not do this should at least do the above-mentioned in order to create team spirit at the practice.

Chapter 6

Rewarding and Increasing Staff Motivation

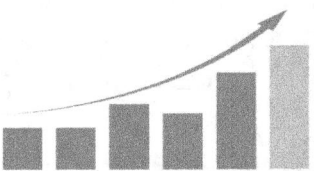

Remunerating Practice Staff

This is undoubtedly one of the most charged and explosive issues at dental practices. There is almost no dental practice owner who does not hesitate when it comes to the question, "How much should I pay the employees?" In fact, this is a conflict with pre-defined explosive interests: employees want to earn as much as possible and the practice owner wants to reduce expenses as much as possible.

As if this is not enough, the dilemma of the salary level for workers involves many emotions – the workers feel that they deserve more and the owner, on the other hand, feels that he is paying too much. The result is that the receptionist's girlfriend tells her that she's getting paid one dollar more per hour at another practice, which is enough to trigger this explosive volcano.

On the other hand, we should remember that workers who do not feel they are getting the salary they deserve will be resentful, and where there are disgruntled employees, success does not exist. Hence, this conflict must not occur and if it does, it must be dealt with immediately. I know too many practices where wage conflict is continuously alive and well. The worker asks for a wage increase, the practice owner chooses to postpone the answer longer and longer, this causes a decline in the worker's motivation, who (instinctively) puts less effort into their work, which also leads to a decline in the revenues and profitability of the practice.

It is important to clarify that this does not mean that the bitter workers who do not receive the salary they think they deserve will not answer the phone or will shout at the customers. In most cases, it will be difficult to tell that they are resentful, but naturally, they will not exert themselves or contribute beyond what is necessary, and that is precisely the difference between mediocrity and success. The difference between the output of a disgruntled employee and that of a satisfied employee are extremely significant.

Nevertheless, it is clear that not every time workers claims they want a raise should the owner of the practice comply in order to avoid conflict. Before thinking about how to reward the workers, the connection between the workers' wages and their motivation and its impact on practice performance must be examined.

How to Reward the Practice's Staff

The question of how to optimally reward the practice's staff has no unequivocal answer. On this issue, there are more grey areas rather than black or white ones – the level of salary per employee is mostly a matter of the administrative approach of the practice owner. The only thing that is clear and absolute in determining the salary is that the owner of a practice is required to pay employees a salary above the minimum wage and to provide them with all the benefits required by law. As mentioned, everything beyond this is a matter of approach.

The wage approach that I advocate and have found to be successful is based on four principles:

1. **Low wages, low performance** – As noted, low wages cause low motivation and worse, the absence of good workers from the practice. Quality employees are not low-wage workers, and as I mention in another chapter of this book, "If you pay peanuts, monkeys will work for you." The result is that low wages for employees may save some expenses, but on the other hand, they prevent the practice from reaching the high sales turnover it could reach if more quality workers were to be employed.

   Every practice's goal is to reach the highest sales turnover possible (realizing its potential). This can only be done with quality employees who are satisfied with their salary. Therefore, it's better to pay a little more than usual and reach maximum sales cycles than to pay low wages and maintain a minimal sales cycle.

   Therefore, if, for example, the standard wage in the industry ranges from X to Y, it is better that you offer wages that are closer to the top (Y) rather than the bottom (X). Believe me, what guides me here is the best interests of the practice, not the employee's welfare. As stated, the equation is very simple: high wages attract quality employees, who lead the practice to good sales cycles, and vice versa.

2. **Dissatisfied? Not with us!** – An iron rule in compensation of employees is not to employ people who are not happy with their salary. As mentioned above, employees of this kind do not invest all of their energy and thus cannot contribute as much to the practice as they potentially could. Hence, my approach is very simple: either you pay the employee the salary they ask for, or you should find someone else to fill the job for the salary you want to pay. As noted, employing a disgruntled employee does not pay off. It's not personal – employees have the right to ask for the salary they think they deserve, and you have the right to decide whether you are willing to pay the requested salary or not. If you have a better alternative, make it a reality. But if you cannot get a better employee while paying less, then raise the worker's wage with the understanding that these are the rules of the game and that this move may eventually increase your sales cycles.

3. **Do the workers want to earn more? No problem, they should improve their performance!** – There must be a direct link between the practice's performance and the salary of the practice staff. This is especially true of the practice's employees who are involved in closing the treatment plans and in the collection: the receptionist and the practice manager. There should not be a practice with low or mediocre performance paying high wages. Therefore, wages must be made up of a base that will enable security and peace of mind for the employee, as well as bonuses for increased turnover at the practice. **(I will expand on this in the next chapter, "Increasing the Motivation of the Practice's Staff.")**

This method is excellent because the workers can never claim that they are not being paid enough. The practice owner can always say, "You can earn more – it's up to you. Improve the practice's performance and your salary will increase accordingly." Let's guess what will happen next.

4. **Medical Staff Salaries** – When dealing with the salaries of the practice's staff it is common to consider the salary of assistants, receptionists, and practice managers without paying attention to the high expenses that are the dentists' salaries. Many

practice owners fail when it comes to contracts with dentists, and this failure may be expressed in spending a great deal of money over the years. Of course, you have to reward the dentists enough that they come to work with motivation to give patients the best care; however, you should avoid some common mistakes in dentist compensation.

The first and most common mistake is the method of offering the dentist hourly wages. This makes no sense for a number of reasons: First, if there is a cancellation the dentists are compensated for the time even though they did not perform the work. Second, the dentists are not interested in producing a high output because they earn by the hour and not according to the treatments they perform. The above reasons often create conflicts between the owner and the dentists and therefore there is no reason to work with this method.

The most popular method of compensation – dentists' compensation according to a percentage of the cost of the treatments they carry out – suffers from significant shortcomings. In practices where prices are relatively high, the dentists' compensation is very high. By the way, in practices that charge high prices, the expenses are usually also higher than the standard (rent, etc.) and therefore there is no economic sense in rewarding dentists according to this method.

Another disadvantage of this method is that in cases where the practice gives a discounted rate as in the case of an extensive treatment plan, the dentist's compensation is particularly low, and this may create a conflict between them and the practice.

Therefore, the most recommended and fair compensation method for both the practice and the dentists is "reward according to procedure." According to this method, the dentists are allocated a fixed amount for each procedure they perform at the practice, regardless of how much the customer paid or whether they received a discount, and regardless of the practice's prices. By the way, here, too, it is worth determining a reward for the dentists in order to create high motivation and loyalty toward the practice. This method is also recommended for rewarding dental hygienists.

Increasing the Motivation of the Practice's Staff

One of the most interesting discussions in the marketing world is the question, *Who has the greater influence on the company's success – the customers or the employees?* I'll go straight to the bottom line: customers have a strong impact on the business success of the company, but employees are more influential! Why? Because if employees are not satisfied, customers will not be happy either. It sounds funny and even simplistic but in fact, this is a significant strategic change in perspective.

It used to be theorized that in order to succeed in business, customer satisfaction must be achieved; today, in business theory there is a lot more emphasis on a change in priorities: the workers must be satisfied first.

All the recommendations presented in this book, which are intended to improve the practice's performance, cannot be implemented without a high level of motivation in the practice's staff. A leading concept in the business world says, *Behind every successful business there is a motivated team.* The same applies to your dental practice. Behind every successful practice, there is a highly motivated, successful team with a desire for the practice to succeed.

A highly motivated team will fight for every treatment plan and go after the issue of collection, they will provide good service to customers so as not to lose them, and will do everything to prevent customers and tasks from falling between the cracks. They will increase customer numbers and initiate marketing activities to recruit customers, as well as hold on to existing ones and manage the practice as if it were their private business. Of course, on the other hand, a team of workers without motivation will come to work and do just enough to justify their salary.

The staff's level of motivation is in your hands. Many books have been written on the issue of increasing motivation and developing team spirit among the staff. Most of them contain obvious advice such as a pat on the employee's back and employee participation in decision making, instead of giving them instructions to implement.

I choose to focus on two main ways in which you can increase the motivation of your practice staff. The first is emotional and the second is material.

1. **Appreciation** – Although people go to work mainly to earn a living, nowadays it's not enough. Appreciation is a basic need and exists from childhood. Incidentally, it is actually the good workers who look for encouragement, and the appreciation they receive pushes them to continue to succeed. Therefore, the practice owner must continually praise and appreciate the work of the practice staff in order to increase motivation and keep pushing the practice forward.

   Unfortunately, in practice the opposite is true. As part of my marketing consultation, one of the most common complaints I hear from dental practice employees is, "The practice owner does not appreciate what we do."

   There are those who feel very comfortable with making complements while others are not as comfortable with this. It is, of course, a matter of character. However, it is important that every practice owner be aware of the importance of expressing appreciation to the practice staff in order to increase motivation.

   So how do you do this? Very simple: was it a very successful month in terms of sales? Express appreciation to the practice manager by saying, "Well done, you did an amazing job!" – even if the successful work is rewarded with financial bonuses. Financial compensation does not replace emotional reward. Did the receptionist handle a client's complaint exceptionally well? Say, "Well done, you showed incredible patience and I really appreciate it."

   Of course, appreciation should also be expressed in other areas, such as showing tolerance when someone makes a mistake, or expressing understanding and empathy for personal needs such as vacations, absences, early departures from work, etc. It's not easy to motivate a team; it's like any relationship. You have to invest and invest in order to preserve this delicate relationship and make it work. On the other hand, you must remember that a practice cannot succeed without a loyal team that truly wants its success.

2. **Rewards according to meeting goals** – If you continue to reward employees the way you have been, in other words, with a fixed monthly salary, you will most likely continue to receive the same sales averages – approximately 15%.

   However, if you succeed in turning the practice staff into "business partners" and give them bonuses when there is an increase in sales, they will exert a lot more effort in order to increase the sales cycle. It is important to note that the distribution of bonuses relates mainly to employees connected directly to sales at the practice, such as the practice manager or the receptionist (and in some cases also the assistant). As for hygienists, there are other ways to increase their salaries, and dentists' salaries will increase with an increase in the practice's activity.

Another point that is important to clarify is that a more effective method for motivating employees than monetary compensation has not yet been invented. With all due respect to the pat on the back (don't give it up) and the good word, if your team knows they can add a few more hundred dollars and perhaps even more to their monthly salary, they will do anything to get the bonus; once they taste the bonus they will want it every month.

How does the method work? It's very simple; take the average sales of the last 12 months. Add 15% for cyclical fluctuations. On each increase of the amount, upon receipt, reception staff and the support team are rewarded with a certain bonus.

What is the optimal bonus? Every practice has to run its own calculations and weigh parameters such as: How many employees are rewarded? Is the sales cycle large or small relative to the market? How much does each employee work? And differences in seniority between employees. In any case, it is necessary to establish a simple and clear formula for the practice owner as well the employees.

Another important point for the success of this move is that the bonus not be too high, in order to keep the practice profitable from the increase in sales. A bonus that is too low, on the other hand, will not create the desired motivation among the staff. The bonus amount should be within a reasonable range.

For example, a practice whose sales turnover is $100,000 a month should adjust the bonus so that if sales increase by $70,000, the two receptionists and two assistants will receive an additional $700 per salary. The total investment in bonuses will be $2,800 but on the other hand, the practice's sales will grow – thanks to the motivation – by $70,000! In this way both the employees and the practice will benefit from this process.

Additionally, the bonuses should be distributed on a sliding scale. A practice that achieves sales of $100,000 on average should set the bar at $250,000 or $300,000 per month and hand out significant bonuses for these cycles in order to challenge the team to reach particularly high sales cycles. You will not believe what happens to employees when goals are set for them and they are rewarded for meeting them.

Incidentally, this program could also work for a practice with a single dentist and an assistant who is also responsible for marketing and administration. For example, you can decide with the assistant that for every increase in sales above the annual average of $10,000 she/he will receive $450 in addition to their salary.

In order for the program to succeed, another matter must be observed. Once a week, let's say on either every Monday or Thursday, the sales cycle must be updated. The figure should hang at the receptionist's desk so you can see where the practice stands in relation to the targets you have set. The purpose of this is to motivate the team to reach the target and surpass it in order to get the bonus. A team of employees which feels close to attaining the target (even when the target is far away) receives an incentive to conduct an efficient collection process, to work hard to obtain every treatment plan, give better service to customers, initiate marketing activities in order to increase sales, etc. – and that's exactly what the practice needs.

The method of encouraging employees through bonuses is the most popular method used in today's business world. Some will say that using this method in a dental practice is taking it a step too far. I think otherwise; there is nothing wrong with using this method in a dental practice. The medical work will not be less professional if the practice is conducted in a more businesslike manner. The practice staff performs many activities during the workday and without incentives and working towards goals, things will not work as well and be less profitable.

By the way, there are quite a few practices that do not disclose sales cycles to employees, in which case this method cannot be used. I have never understood these practices' concern about employees knowing the sales cycle – after all, the same team also deals with the collection of funds, so they have an idea of the practice's income. However, most importantly, it is a great blow to motivation; a staff that is not aware of the sales cycle at any given moment is like football players not knowing the score. The result of the game, i.e., the monthly goal, is the main engine for motivation and so it should be in every practice.

Chapter 7

"Personal Branding" of Dentists

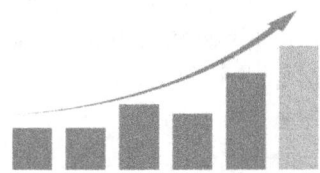

The dentist's behavior towards the client during treatment is probably the most important aspect of dental practice marketing. As detailed in the previous chapters, the most important parameter for customers when choosing a dentist or practice is the dentist's level of professionalism. Since, as I have shown, customers do not have the ability or the objective tools with which to measure the professionalism of the dentist, they will examine, judge, and choose according to the dentist's conduct towards them.

In the many observations I have performed on the conduct of dentists during treatments, I witnessed a few strange scenes that do not add – to put it mildly – to the credit and professional positioning of the dentist in customers' eyes. Consider the cellphone saga: quite a few dentists answer their phones during treatment. At best, they let their assistant answer but continue to negotiate with the representative of the implants company on the line: "Tell him I don't accept the price he sent over" quickly becomes, "Give me the phone for a minute." Before you know it, we have forgotten all about Mr. Smith (who has invested hundreds of dollars here) lying on the unit with his mouth open, and with a lot of free time. He hears the conversations, observes, judges, and writes the dentist off as unprofessional.

On the other hand, I have also encountered quite a few dentists who know how to interact well with customers and position themselves as highly professional. These dentists understand the importance of their behavior and its influence on their professional image. They deposit their cellphone at the reception desk at the beginning of the shift, receiving reports only between treatments. It is no accident that these dentists are usually also the most successful.

The poor conduct of dentists in relation to patients is probably due to the great enemy of most dentists: professional burnout. Dentistry is one of the most demanding and exhausting professions in the market today. A dentist sees dozens of patients a day, each with different and unique needs.

The dentist must maintain a high level of concentration during all working hours and be precise to the millimeter. And if this is not enough, most of the activity takes place in the early and late evening – when the dentist also requires time for his relationships on the family front. In simple terms, as one dentist put it, "I feel like I'm working on an assembly line."

The issue of burnout is something every dentist must consider and look out for. Coping with burnout must be conducted on two levels: the first, the mental aspect – taking vacations, taking on interesting hobbies, etc. The second, and most important, is awareness – if the dentists understands that present and future professionalism depends on how they relate to the patients, they will adopt professional conduct.

In fact, there is a deep conflict within the dentist's conduct toward their patients. On the one hand, dentists are in a situation of an "assembly line" job – they have already seen ten customers, with ten more to go until the end of the shift – and on the other hand is the individual patient. For the dentist this is the 11th customer out of 20, but from the customer's point of view, this is the only and most important appointment.

With most of the dentist's business success depending on existing clients (who will continue to be their customers, and recommend them to their acquaintances), there is no doubt which side should adapt to the other. You guessed it, the dentists and all of the practice staff must adapt to the clients and give them the feeling that they are the one and only. Forgive the cynicism, but otherwise they will have no one to give this feeling to.

In fact, there are several elements that the dentist needs and can achieve by appropriate conduct in front of the customer during treatment.

1. **Strengthening his/her professional image in the customer's eyes.**

2. **Strengthening his/her image as empathic and gentle during treatment.**

3. **Developing personal relationships (within the boundaries of good taste, of course) with customers.**

4. **Directing maximum attention to the customers and their needs.**

How do you do this? In the following way:

1. **General preparation for the workday** – If you arrive at the practice about 30 minutes before the beginning of the workday, the entire shift may look different. You should use this time to sit with the receptionist and assistant and go over the list of customers arriving today; make sure that the final lab work has arrived, go through the patients' files – what treatments you are performing today, the collection status, etc. Such preparation may prevent many problems on the job over the course of the day. If you come in at the same time as the first patient or worse, after him – and unfortunately, this is common with quite a few dentists – complications and problems are guaranteed.

   I had the privilege of observing an amazing practice with a devoted staff. The entire staff makes sure to arrive at the practice an hour before work began. The head dentist, who owns the practice, delivers a short talk and afterwards they have a briefing and preparation for the workday. They drink coffee, eat croissants, and only then welcome the first customer. This practice is run so well that their main problem is the appointment load.

2. **Customers love it when you take an interest in them** – Sales experts make a point of recording details of personal information about their customers so that they can conduct a small talk and create closeness. Be sure to record personal details about the customer in the treatment file such as, *Works in the air conditioning business; planning a wedding for his son in March*. Initiate small talk with the customers immediately upon their arrival – customers love it when interest in their well-being and that of their family is expressed and they feel most comfortable talking about subjects they understand.

   Imagine how good a customer would feel if you welcomed him as follows: "Hello Mr. Smith, how are you? How was your son's wedding? By the way, I wanted to ask you about my air conditioning; it's been giving me some trouble." It should be noted here that there is no intent of developing a personal relationship with the client, but rather creating personal closeness and sympathy. It is more likely that customers will feel comfortable when being treated by a dentist who they feel generates compassion and openness.

3. **Prepare for the client's arrival** – It takes exactly two minutes. Before the clients come in (returning after the first visit), go over their file: their first name,

the treatments they have had so far, what is planned for the current treatment, and so on.

In this way, when they sit down you can call them by their first name (this is their favorite sound) and brief them on what was done, what you are doing today, and what remains to be done as part of the treatment: "Mr. Smith, last time we measured the crown on your back tooth, and today we will perform two extractions in preparation for the implant. At the next session we will finish the front tooth crown."

This action achieves two significant things: First, the dentist addresses and eases the client's uncertainty by informing them of the stage of the treatment plan that is going to be performed. In addition, the client understands that there is progress in the treatment, not just in the payments. Second, the dentist communicates to the customers that he/she has prepared for them and that they are not just another customer on the assembly line. I swear to you, I heard the following with my own ears at one of my observations at a practice: when a client entered the treatment room the dentist asked him, "So what are we doing today?" This is not a mistake – the dentist asked the client what to do today, not the other way around. In other words, the dentist gave the client the following message: "I didn't prepare for you; you're just one of many clients, and in fact, you shouldn't have come in." It's not difficult to guess what this conduct does to a client's perception of the dentist's professionalism.

The Dentist's Conduct during Treatment

1. **"Careful, the injection stage has arrived!"** – An average dentist sees giving a shot to a client as a trivial matter, but for the average customer it is a significant matter and for some it is also very traumatic. I'm not exaggerate when I say that in fact, the injection stage is the most crucial moment in the customer's relations with the dentist. We must remember that in this instant the clients are most judgmental; I have heard patients say, "My dentist is amazing – you do not feel the injection at all."

Performing a gentle injection, with advance warning and an apology – "I'm sorry but I'll have to hurt you a bit. I will try to do it as gently as possible" – may grant the dentist many credit points, both professional and personal. Hence, to be sensitive and gentle at this stage is to gain valuable points.

Incidentally, I've come across a smart dentist who had banned the entire practice staff from using the word 'injection' in the presence of patients.

2. **Quiet, we're working here** – Some dentists prefer to remain silent during treatment in order to concentrate on the work or maybe think about their next ski vacation. Other dentists prefer to talk to clients during treatments and share every step and action they take. Both options are problematic – on the one hand, silence on the part of the dentist and assistant create a feeling of distress, and on the other hand, a very detailed explanation of every action performed may bother the client.

Therefore, a balance must be found in order to prevent the clients from the uncomfortable feeling of *I wonder what is going on in my mouth*. It is useful to share with them from time to time during the treatment, "Mrs. Green, I am now clearing up the inflammation that caused you pain." Of course, this also depends on the client's personality.

3. **Where is your concentration?** – I have come across quite a few dentists who like to talk to the assistant during treatment. The assistant tells the dentist about the family event that took place last night, the dentist shares doubts about the new dentist that he is interested in employing, and so on. Oops, we forgot something again – there's someone on the chair, her name is Mrs. Green, and she's the client who entrusted you with her health care as well as hundreds or even thousands of dollars from her pocket.

Mrs. Green, who has nothing to do during the treatment except listen to the dentist and assistant, thinks the assistant is gossipy and petty because he has only said negative things about the event, and that the dentist is stingy because he is not willing to pay the new dentist the salary he asked for even though he is great at his job.

However, there is an even more problematic matter: Mrs. Green thinks, and rightly so, that not all attention is dedicated to treating her, which could harm the quality of treatment – *How can he talk and joke and be precise about the root canal?* With such behavior, you will have a customer who is jumpy and anxious throughout the treatment instead of being relaxed about having placed themselves in your hands. Therefore, it is recommended that you leave the chitchat with the assistant, the phone calls with the implant provider, troubleshooting for the staff, and all the other issues that distract you from the client for another time. The customers are here and they deserve all of your attention.

4. **Message Package** – Treatment time is a good time to convey positive messages to the customer related to your professionalism and competitive advantages. It is worthwhile to gradually and gently convey the messages according to relevance, but in any case, you must remember: if you do not tell the customers that you are a professional, how else will they know?

   Here is an example of messages that express innovation and strengthen your professional image, which you can pass on to the client during treatment: "All the recent studies I have read show clearly that..." Or, "At the last conference I attended in the United States I presented a similar case to yours and in terms of the conclusion, is pretty clear that..." Or, "Do not worry, over my 17 years of experience with dental implant treatment I have come across much more complicated cases than yours which ended successfully."

5. **Relaxing the patients** – It is worth checking from time to time that everything is okay with the clients. Of course, it is obligatory to inform them at the beginning of treatment that if they feel pain they should raise their hand and treatment will be stopped immediately; you are giving them a sense of control, which is very important. Saying things like, "Is everything okay?" Or, "We will be done in ten minutes." Or, "If you wish to take a break let me know" may significantly improve the customer's confidence in you.

6. **Humor** – A sense of humor is an asset for the dentist. Even if you're not a comedian by nature, you may want to have a number of jokes or comments prepared that will create a positive atmosphere during treatment. Of course, you should choose the right jokes (beware of sexist and racially inappropriate ones) so that they will not offend the customer and backfire on you.

7. **A few more points that a dentist should pay attention to:**

   A. If Mr. Smith was admitted late for treatment due to delayed appointments or an unexpected emergency appointment, he should receive an apology. He will appreciate it very much and show understanding.

B. There is something nice about the dentist going out to the waiting area and inviting the client to the treatment room. In this case, he/she can also see what the situation in the waiting room is and will also be perceived as hospitable. After all, the client is actually your guest.

C. At the end of each treatment, suggest that the clients call if they have any questions. Don't worry; they will not hurry to call, but will appreciate the invitation.

D. Do not economize when it comes to an attractive dentist's coat. If you wear a faded coat with an ink stain in the pocket, you will be perceived by the customer accordingly. In order to come across as a professional dentist it is preferable to wear a white coat rather than a green uniform, even though the latter is more comfortable.

E. Charm the clients – Give them something they did not expect and which is not part of the treatment. For example, clean the nicotine smear on their front tooth; give them tips on how to maintain oral hygiene such as gargling with salt water; or give them free mouthwash (no samples!), a good toothbrush, and so on.

F. Do not forget to explain to the customers how important it is to get their plaque removed as part of preventing future dental problems. If they do not come in for this, you may lose contact with them. The responsibility for this is on you and not the hygienist since the clients are more receptive to your messages.

Chapter 8

Assistants' Conduct toward the Dentist and Clients

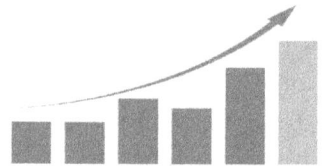

During my many visits to dental practices, I have encountered two main types of assistants: The first are the assistants who perform their role in the strict sense of the word; they help the dentist mix the ingredients and hand him instruments during treatment. The second type, in addition to their basic role, help the dentist with breathing life into the practice, and help the patients get through the treatment. The first type of assistant is a dentist's aide while the other kind is an important marketing asset to the practice.

The assistant's role should be primarily helping clients get through the treatments in a positive way and only afterwards as a dentist's aide. The assistant's status at the practice also depends on their personality, but mainly on the way that the dentist sees the role. Dentists, who treat assistants as an aide and pay them accordingly, will be assisted with no initiative and with minimal contribution to the practice – or, as the saying goes: "If you pay peanuts, monkeys will work for you." On the other hand, dentists who pay assistants adequate wages and bestow challenging responsibilities on them will experience a lively spirit and an improvement in customers' feelings at the practice.

Assistants can take on many roles and help clients through the treatments in a more pleasant manner because they are close to both the dentist and the client during the course of the treatment. The assistant is exposed to all the information about the client, both on the personal level and the details of the treatment plan. Additionally, it is easier and more convenient for customers to communicate with the assistant than with the dentist. The assistant speaks their language; they have medical knowledge and experience, and in many cases can act as a "translator" for the dentist. Sometimes clients are in such awe of the dentist that they feel more comfortable with the assistant.

One of the practices I consulted initiated a brilliant move. For every patient who entered, an assistant who served as a liaison between him or her and the practice was assigned for the duration of the treatment plan. Clients received an explicit statement from the start, during the presentation of the treatment plan: "If you chose us for dental care, our assistant Linda will be your liaison. If you have any medical question you are welcome to call us and talk to Linda."

The fact that customers have a contact person, who will answer their medical questions for any length of time during the treatments, significantly improves their feelings and reduces uncertainty. When this fact is made clear to customers at the stage of presenting the treatment plan, it may promote the client's decision to perform the treatment with your practice.

Customers have all kinds of concerns and 'light' medical questions that bother them before and during the treatment such as, "Will I have to walk around without teeth after the extraction? Will I have to wait after the bone transplant?" The clients will not want to bother the dentist with every question they have and are also a little afraid that their questions will sound silly, but on the other hand they don't feel comfortable asking the receptionist since they are not familiar with their file on a medical level. Therefore, the assistants are the most appropriate people to fill this role and they also have the most access to a dentist.

The assistant's behavior should convey the following messages during treatments:

1. **Dear customer, don't worry – you come first!** – It is highly recommended that the assistant arrange the tray and replace the drinking glass only after the next customer sits in the unit. If there is anything customers are afraid of its drinking from a glass someone else used, or god forbid, be treated with instruments that have already been in someone else's mouth.

2. **A customized practice** – The dentist and assistant should adapt to the clients rather than the other way around. That way, clients will feel the most comfortable and that's exactly how we want them to feel. For example, if there is a TV on the ceiling, the assistant, as the host, should give the remote control to the client and invite them to watch the channel of their choice. Or if the air conditioning is on, ask whether the temperature is pleasant.

   Since we are already hosting and customizing to accommodate the clients, one of the suggestions I make to practices is that in each treatment room there be a selection of four or five popular types of music to choose from. Before starting treatment, the assistant should ask the client, "What would you like to hear from our selection?" In other words, *We are completely adapting ourselves to you, and not vice versa.* There is no better feeling than this for customers. I recommend you try this at any practice!

3. **Yes, Doctor!** – In the presence of patients, the assistant must address the dentist with the title "Doctor" only. There are assistants who have worked with the dentist for many years and a sign of their friendship is calling the dentist by his/her first name in front of the client. This does not contribute to improving the client's perception of the dentist's professionalism; on the contrary. In general, it is good to maintain some distance between the dentist and the clients.

4. **Is everything okay?** – During treatment, the assistant should indeed help the dentist, but also show concern about the welfare of the client. It is highly recommended that they occasionally reassure the customer and make sure everything is fine: "Is everything okay?" Or, "Do you want to rinse your mouth?" Or, "Are you comfortable?" And so on. Such concern may significantly improve the customer's wellbeing. Even light touches on the shoulder may give the customers the feeling that they are in good hands.

Chapter 9

The Dental Hygienist's Conduct and Increased Productivity

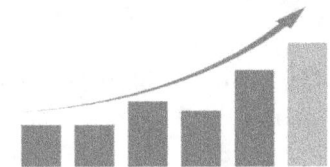

The dental hygienist's work is one of the most important contributors to the success of the dental practice, if only because their main function is the retention of customers. A client who makes sure to go to the practice every six months for a cleaning is a customer who, when in need of dental care, will probably go to that practice. Additionally, if some of his acquaintances ask him if he knows of a good dentist, chances are that he will not hesitate to recommend the practice.

The math is very simple – the more customers come in for regular treatments, the more active customers the practice will have who make recommendations to their acquaintances. Of course, the more active customers are the more active the practice's cash register will be.

However, the reality in most dental practices is much less optimal. In fact, for most customers, in most practices, plaque removal is not done every six months. Let's conduct a simple calculation: in a practice which has existed for more than ten years and served thousands of clients, if the hygienist had performed a cleaning every six months for each of the practice's clients (or at least most of them), the practice should be completely booked for many months in advance. However, as noted, this is not the reality in most practices.

There is also good news: this fantasy can become a reality. I have encountered some practices where the reality is sunny and most customers do come in for a cleaning every six months. This is not by chance; all of these practices work according to the method I suggested to them and reached the desired result: a very lively turnover in the hygienist's chair. However, before I get to how to do it, we should understand what makes most practices fail in such an important area.

In fact, the average dental hygienist faces two major problems:
1. Many clients are not aware of the importance of plaque removal and its effect on dental health.
2. For many customers, there is no distinction between hygienists – they are perceived as just there to clean teeth.

In order for dental hygienists to achieve high productivity, they and the practice must deal with these two problems.

1. **Many customers are not aware of the importance of plaque removal and its impact on dental health** – Customers think in terms of profit and loss. As long as customers do not understand the importance of the removal, why would they agree to waste their time and money on such a treatment? In contrast, if the clients understand that most dental problems result from accumulation of plaque and that removal may prevent some of them, you can be certain that they will chase the practice in order to set up an appointment on time. This is exactly the reason why people run to the garage when it's time to for their annual servicing: they worry that if they do not take care of the car it will break down, which may be very unpleasant and very expensive.

The primary responsibility for increasing customer awareness about the importance of dental cleaning lays with dentists and not hygienists. For customers, dentists are the authority in the field and therefore their recommendation or diagnosis is of more importance than any other professional's in the practice is. In other words, if customers do not come in for a cleaning at the practice the dentists have failed to raise their awareness of plaque damage.

Imagine a situation in which the client lays in the chair and the dentist tells him, "Mr. Smith, most dental problems are caused by plaque. If you had come in for a cleaning every six months, there is a good chance that we could have avoided this extraction of both teeth from your lower jaw. The cleaning would have both saved your teeth and saved you the hundreds of dollars that you are now spending on implants. For your sake, I hope that you will make regular dental cleaning a priority in the future so that you do not lose any more teeth."

When the customer is presented with a loss that may be caused (or has already been caused) due to not coming in for routine treatment, there is no chance he will not come in once every six months. We have already concluded that customers think in terms of profit and loss. Not surprisingly, in practices where the dental hygienist's appointment book is full for weeks in advance, I see dentists who spend a lot of time raising customer awareness about cleaning. On the other hand, in most other practices dentists do remind the patients about this and do not emphasize the matter.

Therefore, dentists must pay more attention to the transmission of messages to customers about the importance of removing plaque. This is true both in terms of the medical aspect of preventative care and from the business aspect of customer retention.

2. **For many customers, there is no difference between hygienists** – Many customers see the treatment as just a cleaning. Of course, this is not true, but instead of blaming customers, you should ask what the hygienists should do so that customers think otherwise. Note that customers, after the plaque removal, look in the mirror and say, "Wow, such clean teeth!" They do not talk about the plaque that was removed, but about the cleanliness of the teeth. Moreover, if it's just cleaning, then why is it so important who cleans my teeth?

Successful dental hygienists are those who know how to market themselves and their treatments. Without self-marketing, dental hygienists have no chance of winning over loyal customers and filling up the appointment book for months in advance. The hygienist's self-marketing must be conducted on three levels. First, promoting a professional image: "The method of removing the plaque I perform is different from that of other hygienists." The second level is raising awareness: "If you do not make sure to undergo treatment you may be causing damage to your health." The third level is developing personal relationships with customers: "Hi, Mr. Smith, I'm happy to see you! How's your son doing at university?"

One of the most effective solutions for the hygienist is the preparation of a profile page to be distributed to all clients who come to the practice and especially those who come for plaque removal. The main purpose of the profile page is to strengthen the professional image of the hygienists and differentiate them from other dental hygienists. Another purpose is to provide information about the importance of meticulous plaque removal. The profile page should be formatted on quality paper and include pictures of the hygienists. The first part of the page will summarize their education: where they studied, how many years they have been in the field, a brief description of the courses and classes they took, etc. This data is intended to strengthen the professional image of the hygienists. The second part will discuss what removal treatment is meant for and why it is important to make it a priority.

Hygienists who have adopted my advice and prepared an attractive profile page said their professional image greatly improved in the eyes of the customers. For example, customers were impressed to find out that in order to be a dental hygienist you have to study at the dental faculty in a university. It turns out that most customers believe that in order to work as a dental hygienist a quick course is enough, so specifying such a detail on the profile page can do wonders for the hygienist's image. In addition, customers finally realize what plaque is and how much damage it can cause their teeth if they do not receive treatment according to the recommended frequency – that is, every six months.

Telemarketing

In order for the hygienists to work at full capacity and for your customers to arrive in a regular manner to visit you and the hygienist, you need a telemarketer at the practice. The practice's receptionists cannot do the telemarketing work very well because they are overloaded with the demanding and overwhelming work at the practice such as reminder calls, contact with the lab, collection, shifts, and so on.

Therefore, if the receptionist calls Mr. Smith in order to make an appointment for the dental hygienist and he cannot talk and asks to be contacted later, this may not happen. Or if Mr. Smith tells the receptionist that he is not sure he needs plaque removal and that everything is fine with him, it is not obvious that the receptionist will have the time to tell him about the importance of removal, and so on.

On the other hand, if there are telemarketers at the practice, all they do is reach out to people about removal and periodic checkups and have the time to call customers back and, if necessary, give them a lecture on the importance of plaque removal. The best hours for telemarketing are from 4 PM to 8 PM, but you can also have a day or two of morning shifts since there are customers who are comfortable dealing with these things in the morning. This negligible half-time expense could bring in a lot of money for the practice, dental treatments, and the accompanying treatments that the clients will perform when they come to receive treatment for removal. Most importantly, you will have more active customers who regularly visit the practice and become its ambassadors.

Combining removals with dental examinations

To maximize the hygienists' treatments, you should accustom clients to the fact that this takes place together with a dentist's examination. Dental hygiene treatment should be scheduled at the same time that the head dentist in the practice has a shift, and thereby achieve two important things: First, if the clients complain about something specific such as, "My tooth hurts when I drink something cold" they can immediately see the dentist and perform an x-ray as well as decide on a course of treatment. Secondly, achieving routine checkups and strengthening the patient's relationship with the dentist: "Hey, how are your parents doing? Send them my regards." In addition, the patients receive preventive dental care.

Clients who combine a dental hygiene appointment and an examination also feel that they are getting more value from their visit. Incidentally, an important tactical matter should be considered: it is worth arranging short dental appointments for a dentist working the parallel shift, rather than serious surgical treatments, so that the dentist will have the ability to maneuver between the work and fitting in customers for a brief examination if necessary.

Chapter 10

Pricing Strategy for Treatments

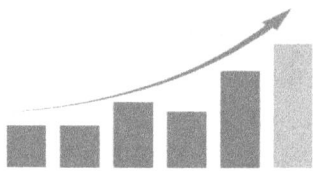

I have met very few dentists who stand behind the prices he/she charges for treatments 100%. Some dentists debate whether to raise the prices and the others debate whether it is worthwhile to lower the prices. In most cases, the dilemma becomes more intense after a customer complains about the high prices, or alternatively, when the accountant presents the practice owner with the worn-out bottom line and unprofitable annual report.

Determining the optimal price for practice treatments can be simple only when the practice staff understands what the practice has to offer and what your main market segment is. One thing is clear – there must be a correlation between the two things. In order to determine the correct price level for the dental practice, you must first define who the main target audience is. **Mercedes**, for example, offers products of very high quality and targets an upper market segment; therefore, it is natural that the prices of its products are high. **Daewoo**, on the other hand, offers products of lower quality and targets a lower market segment and therefore its product prices are accordingly low. **Mazda** and **Toyota** offer good quality cars and appeal mainly to mid-market clients, therefore, the prices of cars are medium-high.

The same business logic that operates in the car industry and other market sectors also works in the dental market. The dental market is also divided into lower, middle, and upper market segments. Every practice must decide which segment it is interested in targeting and offer the types of treatments and quality level appropriate to that segment, and of course price the treatments accordingly. A practice that has not decided to whom it wants to appeal and what it offers will not be able to price its services in the optimal manner. Before you decide which segment you want to target, you may want some data about the various market segments and their characteristics.

1. **The lower market segment** – This is not a small part of the population. This segment earns minimum wage. Its purchasing power is low and as a result, its sensitivity to prices is very high. This market segment favors low-priced products and services and, accordingly, is satisfied with poor quality. This market segment shops at markets and cheap chain stores, and travels in cheap cars or by public transport. This market segment usually neglects its teeth, has no choice but to seek out the cheapest practices, is satisfied with cheaper treatments such as dentures, and prefers bridges to implants. However, because it a matter of health, a certain part of this market will prefer treatment by quality dentists even though the prices are higher.

2. **The middle market segment** – This segment earns an average wage, drives a family car, goes on vacations, and shops at chain stores that provide a shopping experience even though they are a bit more expensive than others are. A large part of this segment pays a mortgage and fights a month-end overdraft, but loves the good life and does not compromise on quality and pampering. This segment is sensitive to prices but also to quality – they will not buy the cheapest product or service but will consider it using quality data.

   Middle-market consumers are considered smarter than lower market consumers are. They know how to conduct market surveys and Google their options before deciding on a dental implant. This segment is willing to pay medium-plus prices, but also requires good service, quality, and professionalism. The largest part of this segment prefers, and also has the ability, to undergo implantations and expensive dental treatments – especially the 50+ age group, who finished paying their mortgage and managed to save up some money on the side.

3. **The upper market segment** – A significantly smaller segment than the other two, which earns a very high salary and its purchasing power is accordingly high. This segment prefers high-quality services and products and is willing to pay for them. However, this market segment is a lot less attractive than it seems, and there are two main reasons for this. First, this highly courted and demanding market segment that expects quality, service, and professionalism that are sometimes beyond what can be provided. In addition, this smart market segment conducts in-depth market research, which makes it not so easy to win over.

We have seen, then, that determining prices is directly related to the market segment that the practice targets. If the practice decides to go after a specific market segment, it should price its treatment accordingly. No less importantly, offer the segment the quality of the care and service that corresponds with these prices. Those who choose to deal with the lower market segment will offer low prices but also will not invest in luxury design and instead use cheap materials so that they can offer treatments at a low price.

There are a number of other issues that affect how prices are determined for treatment:

The Competition's Prices – As a practice owner, you should be familiar with the market price level (through simple industrial espionage) so that you can position yourself correctly in relation to competitors. A good starting point for this is the prices in public dental practices. Roughly, it can be said that these practices are mainly directed at the middle and low market segments, and offer low to medium prices. If you are targeting this market segment, your prices should be equal or 10-20% higher. In any case, prices of private medicine directed at the mid-market should be higher than public medicine. As an analogy, public medicine is a cafeteria, private medicine is a restaurant, and the prices shift accordingly.

If you appeal to lower or higher market segments, prices should vary accordingly. Another important point of reference is your direct competitors. If you are a specialist in oral rehabilitation and there is another dentist with the same specialty in your vicinity from whom you know customers also receive a proposal for a treatment plan, it is worth keeping your prices in the same range unless you have unique competitive advantages that justify higher prices.

Perceived value – Certain competitive advantages may affect the prices of treatments at the practice. If you are a dentist with a specialization, it is obvious that the prices of your treatments will be higher. It is also considered a competitive advantage if you have many years of experience, if you are a graduate of a prestigious dental school, or if your practice has innovative and unique equipment not found in other practices (microscope, CT, etc.). This also works in the other direction: if you do not have competitive advantages over your competitors, you cannot charge higher prices than they do.

Profitability – In most cases, the practice's treatment costs are higher than perceived. Many dentists focus mainly on calculating the costs of materials, wages, rent, etc., and usually ignore additional costs such as depreciation of the units, costs associated with the studies and training of dentists, and so on, so that many practices finish the month or year with a depleted bottom line.

It is worthwhile to understand that a practice that does not make a profit loses twice: First, the dentists are frustrated by the fact that they do not earn enough and therefore come to work reluctantly. Second, customers do not receive quality dental care because the practice cannot afford to invest in new equipment and materials. Both the practice and the clients lose, and this is a cycle that feeds itself. In many cases, if the practice would work within a price range that is only 10% higher than the current price range, the bottom line would be completely different and would change the dentists and customers' experience. A practice that works without profitability does an injustice to itself and its customers.

By the way, you will find more satisfied customers in practices that are more expensive and vice versa. Therefore, when determining the price it is important to ensure that the price generates sufficient profitability for the practice.

Pricing of leading treatments – While pricing the common treatments it must be considered that in most cases, the customers are an indication of the prices of the other treatments provided at the practice. Customers do not know what the price of a bone transplant or apicoectomy is, but they usually know the price of common treatments such as dental hygiene appointments or a white filling, and from their point of view, if the price of hygiene treatment is high then so are the price of bone transplants or sinus lifts and vice versa.

Therefore, it is very important to be careful with the pricing of the common treatments: white fillings and hygiene care. I know of practices where the price of dental hygienists treatment is very high, but the prices of other treatments are actually low. Guess what the customer thinks? You guessed it – that the treatments are very expensive at this practice.

This method is known as "loss leader" pricing and many companies use it quite often – they price common products very low in order to create the impression that their prices are low, which will enable them to earn high profit margins from the products customers are not familiar with in terms of price. For example, IKEA prices their coffee cups very low and distributes them in strategic locations in the customer's path in the store, in order to produce a perception of low prices. McDonald's sells ice cream at a very low price for the same reason.

Consumer behavior – It is important to clarify that many customers link high price to quality, so in many cases clients will prefer the more expensive offer because, from their point of view, it is probably also better and of higher quality.

For example, a middle market segment customer askes for a treatment plan proposal from three practices. The first practice offers the treatment plan for $2,000; the second offers the same program for $2,800; and the third for $3,300. Which practice has the highest chance of winning the client over?

In terms of consumer behavior, what happens to customers is the following: First, they disqualify the first practice offering the cheapest treatment plan, thinking, *Hmm, it is very suspicious that the price is so low. Perhaps the quality of the materials and treatments is not very high.* Second, it is likely that clients will deliberate between the middle plan and the most expensive plan, when the latter has an advantage over the middle and will be more desirable to them: *If the practice is expensive, it must be good.* Consumers think, especially when it comes to cases where they do not have the ability measure the quality of the service, that the price serves as an indication of quality.

There are two important things to learn from this case: first, you do not want to be the cheapest practice, and the second, expensive pricing is an advantage rather than a disadvantage. An important message that I introduce to practices who receive marketing consultation from me is, "When the client tells you that you are expensive accept it as a compliment, because for him you probably must also be high-quality. If the customer asks why you are cheap, then you should start worrying."

PART THREE

THE ART OF CLOSING TREATMENT PLANS

Chapter 11

The Dentist's Self-Marketing when Meeting with Clients

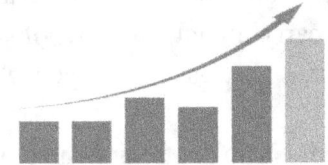

I have spent many hours watching dentists in treatment rooms, during which I discovered that dentists fall into two main categories: some see an encounter with the client as a medical event only, while others succeed in seeing marketing as a familiarizing aspect of the meeting, beyond the medical event.

Dentists, who see an encounter with the client as just a medical event, discuss sinuses, root canals, and other matters in too much detail and forget that they must bring the customers to the decision, "I want only you to take care of me and to hell with the price."

On the other hand, dentists who see an encounter with the client as a marketing event communicate confidence and empathy, as well as the feeling that the client is in the best hands; these dentists will eventually succeed in winning the customer's heart and pocket.

A dentist I taught self-marketing and closing treatment plans told me a story – funny or sad, depending on which side you are on – which illustrates the matter well. A customer came in for a consultation and showed him a proposal for a treatment plan from another dentist. When he reviewed the proposal, he immediately noticed that the dentist who signed the proposal was none other than his best friend from dental school, who had been considered the best student in the faculty. When the customer agreed to start the treatment, even though the price the second dentist offered was 20% higher than was offered to him by the other practice, the dentist could not help himself and asked, "Why didn't you choose to undergo the treatment with the other dentist [that is, the prize student]?" The customer replied, "Are you crazy? Why would I let a shoemaker treat me?"

Of course, the dentist who lost the client is not a shoemaker, more than that; he had been the best student in the department. However, apparently the way he handled the client made him appear as less professional in the customer's mind. The client did not sit next to the dentist in a class in medical school and the way he judged him was solely based on his conduct. In contrast, the dentist I had trained was a lesser student in university but did well in carrying out a number of self-marketing activities with the customer and therefore won his trust and his pocket.

It is important to note that there is no contradiction between the two things. Dentists who self-market to the customer are not less professional. They simply understand the very simple fact that the customers do not have the ability or the tools to know who is a professional dentist and therefore self-marketing becomes necessary. Moreover, dentists who engage in self-marketing have more customers, perform more treatments, gain more experience, and enough resources to catch up on courses, so that eventually they become more professional and more up-to-date. It's a kind of chicken and egg scenario.

The First Encounter with the Client: The Initial Examination

The impression you make on the customers – whether a "shoemaker" or a "professional" – is in fact a mosaic that the clients put together using several actions that you will or will not perform during the first meeting with them, and especially during the initial examination. Be sure that by the end of this exam, the customers will formulate either a solid, positive approach toward you ("He/she is a professional and empathic dentist and I should receive care from him/her and only him/her"), a lukewarm impression ("I should go for a checkup with another dentists"), or even, heaven forbid, a negative impression ("I do not want to be treated by this dentist"). And because perception is reality, it and only it will ultimately affect the client's decision about whether to undergo treatment with you or with another dentist.

Before I deal with the question of what should be done during the initial meeting in order to win the customer's heart and pocket, it is worthwhile to focus on two important points that should guide every dentist in dealing with clients.

The first point is this – the very fact that clients enter your practice says that you earned credit points. In 99% of cases, customers do not walk in because they saw a "Dentist" sign, but rather after collecting positive information such as recommendations from acquaintances. Even if they came thanks to an ad you posted, it means something about it appealed to them – your experience, where you studied dentistry, the location of the practice, or your treatment methods.

The second point is, if customers bother to call for an appointment and come to the dental practice it means that they have a problem and are very interested in solving it – just like no one goes to the garage if their vehicle does not have a malfunction that they need to resolve. Let's compare this to basic consumer behavior: when customers enter the Fashion store **Zara**, this usually indicates two things – one, that they have a positive attitude towards the **Zara** brand (they don't visit every clothing store that exists), and two, they need clothes. The question of whether they will buy and how much depends on what you have to offer and the way you offer it.

Dentists who see customers that come in for consultations as those who come to waste their time treat them as such, and in most cases will probably lose them. On the other hand, dentists who perceive clients in a positive manner will treat them accordingly, and win them over in the end. In the business sense, the dentist's conduct during the initial examination is a self-fulfilling prophecy.

In fact, the initial examination can be divided into four parts:
1. Introduction and creating a sense of closeness to the customer
2. Practiceal examination
3. Diagnosis
4. Presenting alternatives for the treatment plan

Here are some unique "do's and don'ts" for each stage. Apply them for the best chances of winning the customer's heart and pocket:

Step 1 – Introduction and Creating Initial Closeness to the Customer

Studies show that people form a first impression about a new person they have just met, whether positive or negative, in just 40 seconds. This is also true of the initial encounter between a dentist and a client. Sounds unbelievable? Definitely not. If you think about it, it's a kind of blind date. How long does it take the sides to understand that this "isn't it", or that there is actually "something there"? No more than 40 seconds.

During the familiarization stage, you are required to achieve two important things: first, gathering information about the customer before you, and second, eliciting empathy.

How do you do this? In stages and in the following order.

A. **Nice to meet you!** – When you admit the client to the treatment room, you should walk towards them, shake their hand and introduce yourself: "Pleased to meet you, my name is Dr. Jones." See them as guests in your home. Try not to receive them when you are in the middle a phone call, or busy checking the results that just arrived from the lab – and certainly not with your back to them (remember the first 40 seconds?). Be sure to address the customer by their first name – it creates closeness and is their favorite sound in the world.

B. **Eye level** – Be sure to talk to the clients only when they are sitting on the chair and with you sitting in front of them. Talking to the customer when you lean over them and they are seated creates a sense of condescension. Customers like it when you to talk to them at eye level.

C. **Knowledge is power** – Go over the medical questionnaire they filled out in the waiting room and try to gather as much information as possible. Do this gently and not as an interrogation. There are three pieces of information you should know: 1. Where do they live? 2. What do they do for a living? 3. Who referred them to you? (If this data is available.)
This can give you an idea of their financial situation and initial perception of you. For example, if Tom, who performed a complete restoration here and was very pleased, referred them to you, you will know that they already know the price range you offer and that the recommendation they received was very warm or even enthusiastic.

Another piece of important information you should know is where they have been treated in the past, who treated them, whether they were satisfied, and so on. Note that customers will not always be willing to provide you with this information at the first stage and therefore you need to gather the information with sensitivity and their cooperation.

D. Closeness and empathy – Make sure to conduct some chitchat (no more than three minutes) with clients to break the ice and create empathy towards you. The best and shortest way is to find a common interest with them – people feel more comfortable with others who have common interests or shared qualities. If both you and the client like skiing and you're fans of the same football team, they'll feel at ease in your company and prefer to receive care from you.

E. What's bothering you? – Ask the customer, "Tell me, Mr. Smith, what is bothering you?" This is an important question since the clients are about to tell you the most important benefit they wish to get out of the treatment for which they are prepared to pay. If you don't know the main benefit they wish to get out of the treatment, how can you adapt the treatment plan to their needs?

The main benefits of dental care are aesthetics, pain relief, and chewing quality. If the customer says, "Doctor, I'm ashamed to smile," then the main benefit is aesthetics and therefore the proposed treatment plan and messages that you communicate must be focused on aesthetics. The more you focus on the benefit, the more likely you are to win a client over.

An important point: ask the customer what bothers them even before you look in their mouth or examine the x-ray, because you should listen to the customer's needs first, without being affected by your practiceal diagnosis.

Step 2 – Conduct during the practiceal examination

At the examination stage itself you should broadcast two important things: First, you are a professional (because this is the most important thing to customers when choosing a dentist) and second, that you have a gentle touch (because most customers are concerned about dental care). How do you do this? In the following order:

A. Technology – The more technology you use, the more you may be perceived as innovative and professional. You should use an intra-oral camera, glasses with lighting, and so on.

B. Share with the customers – Tell them what you are testing and what you are doing: "Here is the inflammation that caused you trouble at night. I cleaned it out and will give you antibiotics for ten days." Let them know that you know what you are doing and relieve the uncertainty they are experiencing. In any case, there should be no long silences during the examination process; long silences cause distress and even a feeling that you underestimate their ability to understand what is going on.

C. Gentleness – Perform the examination as gently as possible in order to communicate to the client that if they undergo treatment at the practice, they will be treated gently and without pain. Say something like, "I'm sorry, Mr. Smith, I have to hurt you a bit." This sentence should be used before all anesthesia injections. It tells the customer that you are considerate and sensitive.

Step 3 – Presenting a Diagnosis

In presenting the diagnosis, you are required to accomplish two important things: first, to convey the message that you have clearly identified the problem, and second, that the customer understands the diagnosis in general terms.

How do you do this? As follows:

A. Please sit down – Ensure that when the diagnosis is displayed, the client is in a sitting position and you sit face-to-face with them. Lying on the unit and looking at the ceiling will make it difficult for them to understand what you are saying.

B. Be Positive – If you tell the client that their mouth is in a catastrophic state you may put them in a negative mood. They might be angry with themselves for not taking care of their teeth or their family genetics, and may not be in a good enough mood to decide to take care of their teeth and pay quite a bit for this. Therefore, the language should be positive: "Ms. Green, the situation is not as bad as you think. Believe me; a lot of people would be willing to trade places with you." In this way, you will be able to recruit them to the process and make them feel positive about the payment.

C. Simplify – One of the strangest sights I have encountered (and unfortunately there have been many) is the dentist presenting the client with the diagnosis using an x-ray. Dentists are fans of x-rays, but what the customers see is mostly the color black, with white and gray spots. They do not understand that the white and gray sections are inflammation, and the upper part is the sinus. In fact, this does not interest them and they did not come to you for a crash course in dentistry. More than that, looking at the x-ray only confuses them. You should present the x-ray to them but in a nutshell, especially in order to create a professional impression as a dentist, but don't expect them to understand anything from this explanation.

Additionally, you shouldn't talk to them about tooth 26 or tooth 32 – they don't not know what they are ("Wait, Doctor, are you talking about the lower tooth or the upper one?"). This will only add to the uncertainty that they already feel – and the greater the uncertainty, the less likely it is that they will be able to make a decision.

Therefore, it is highly recommended to simplify the diagnosis by using a simple hygienist's dental model, pointing to each tooth and explaining things simply, so that the patient can understand: "Ms. Green, you have an inflammation in this tooth, which is the cause of your pain. This wisdom tooth is pushing on the next tooth and might damage it. These three teeth should be removed, and this tooth and that tooth have cavities."

D. Be decisive – Do not share your doubts about the diagnosis with expressions such as, "I don't know how severe this inflammation is," or, "I'm not sure if it's worth it to pull this tooth," etc. This may position you as indecisive and especially unprofessional. Customers expect solutions from you, not confusion. As far as the customer is concerned, if you're not sure of yourself you are probably not professional enough and therefore it is worth getting an opinion from another dentist.

So if you're not sure about the diagnosis, ask the client for another appointment: "I want to give you a professional answer and will need to examine the x-rays for at least half an hour in order to offer you the best and most professional treatment plan." The customers will appreciate you much more than if you stammer while considering the diagnosis.

E. Create a sense of urgency – If there is no urgency, the customer will postpone implementing the treatment plan. After all, they have more important and fun things to do with the hundreds or thousands of dollars they are supposed to spend on the treatment plan. Therefore, we must create a feeling of urgency, at least for the starting of the treatment – assuming, of course, that there is urgency.

Urgency is considered a situation in which, if the treatment is not done immediately, the situation will only get worse. For example, "Mr. Smith, your wisdom tooth is pushing on the tooth next to it and may destroy it. It is best to remove the wisdom tooth as soon as possible or we will have to remove the second tooth as well." Or, "This tooth requires a normal filling. If we do not do it soon it may turn into a root canal – which will hurt you more and cost more."

It is recommended to mark one or two treatments with a red pen as *Very urgent!* Even if the overall plan is very expensive and the client needs to consult with a partner or banker, they will be able to make an immediate decision to begin the treatment on the two inexpensive stages (an extraction and filling, for example). This sales strategy is called the "foot in the door" method, because instead of trying to open the door all at once, you should first open it only a little and then opening the entire door becomes easier and in most cases turns into a full plan.

It makes a lot of sense. If the customer starts with two small treatments and is satisfied, it is likely that they will decide to carry out the continuation of treatment with you. However, if they only come out with a proposal for an expensive treatment plan, they will probably do a market survey, considering other practices; in such a situation, you should hope that the other practices are less impressive and more expensive than you are.

Step 4 – Presenting alternatives to the treatment plan

In presenting the alternatives, you should achieve two main things: First, the clients must understand the plans and the differences between them. Second, the clients should make a clear decision on what treatment plan they want to undergo.

How do you do this?

A. **More than one plan** – Beyond the fact that the law requires more than one plan to be offered to the client in some countries, in terms of marketing and sales, offering several alternatives (but not more than three!) increases the chances of customers making a decision about one of them. Why? Because it is easier for people to make a decision when faced with a few alternatives. This is why there are no women's clothing stores that sell only black clothes, even though a high percentage of the clothing women prefer is black. In order to buy the black garment they have to see the yellow and red clothes nearby even though they will not buy them. Therefore, you should always present at least one other alternative, even if it is clear to you that the customer will not choose it (for example, prosthetics). If you do not present an alternative, how will the clients be able to compare and make the decision?

B. **Review proposals** – Confused customers do not make a decision. Therefore, you must display the alternatives in a way that is clear and understandable. The initial stage should include a brief and general explanation on alternatives without going into unnecessary details. "Mr. Smith, you have three main treatment options: the first – dentures; the second – dentures on implants; and the third – regular dental implants."

In order to clearly display the alternatives, it is recommended that you use a board hung in the office, high-quality, clean and smooth paper (not the paper on which the instruments are placed, as many dentists do). Clearly write the options: Program A – Dentures, Program B – Dentures on implants, Program C – Regular dental implants.

C. **The decision is yours** – Many dentists fail at this point because they decide which plan the customer should choose and try to lead them to it. The problem is that when trying to lead somebody, they instinctively resist. Customers do not like it when someone else decides for them, and although it is reasonable to assume that they will ultimately adopt your recommendation, they want to feel that the decision was theirs alone.

Another point is the possibility that, for economic or other reasons, the client may not choose the program you tried to promote. They will probably not choose the other plans you suggested, since you probably told them it was the best plan, which means that the other plans are not good enough, or they just do not want to disappoint you.

Therefore, the approach here should be, "Mr. Smith, I presented you with the practiceal diagnosis and treatment options. Deciding what to do is up to you. All the options I have presented you with are good. There is a Subaru, Toyota, and Mercedes – all of them will take you to the destination but it depends on how much pampering and comfort you want along the way and how much you are willing to pay for it."

D. **The method of elimination** – Since the customers find it difficult to decide between three alternatives, it is worthwhile to reduce the dilemma to only two plans: "Mr. Smith, let's go over the alternatives. Are you interested in dentures?" The client may answer, "There is no chance I will get dentures; my friend had them done and he is not satisfied." In such a situation, the client's hesitation is reduced to two programs. Now the situation is simpler: "Okay, Mr. Smith, so we have to choose between the *Toyota* and the *Mercedes*."

E. **Customers love the middle** – Which treatment plan will the customer decide on in the end? The highest probability is that it will be the middle plan, in terms of scope and price (*Toyota*). One of my favorite exercises in the sales workshops I conduct is asking the participants the following question: "You are about to buy a TV and you have three options: a 40-inch screen that costs $1,000, a 52-inch screen that costs $1,500, and a 65-inch screen at $2,500. Which one do you choose?"

Most respondents choose a 52-inch screen (you're welcome to try the exercise at home). The workshop participants are surprised that as soon as the results are announced, I present a page that has been prepared in advance which says, "Customers choose the middle option: a 52-inch screen!" I did not invent the wheel. The TV exercise has been conducted in many studies around the world and it has been proven beyond any doubt that customers love the middle. It is no accident that *Toyotas* and *Mazdas* are the bestselling in the world. What is behind the middle preference? Customers avoid cheap alternatives, fearing that inexpensive means not high-quality, and on the other hand, few of them have the budget to buy the most expensive and the highest-quality, so they feel comfortable with the middle. It is important to make intelligent use of the middle equation. Unfortunately, I have come across too many dentists trying to push the *Mercedes*, and the clients, who prefer the "Toyota treatment," go shopping at another practice.

F. **What's your decision?** – The most important thing in the final stage of presenting alternatives is that you hear the client, and they hear themselves, say which treatment plan they want to undergo. In fact, in order for the client to carry out the treatment plan, they should answer "Yes" to two questions: First – are they interested in choosing plan X presented to them? Second – are they willing to pay the amount that the practice is asking for the treatment? Until the customer answers, "Yes" to the first question – "I want to execute program X," they will not be able to answer "Yes" to the second question – "I am ready to pay the amount needed for it."

Sales and negotiation experts know how to make a clear distinction between the two questions and get a "Yes" to the first question before they bargain with the customers about the price. Why is this so important? Because if you reach the price question before the customers have formulated a decision about which treatment plan they want to carry out, there is no chance in the world that they will say "Yes" to the price and close the plan.

But what to do if customers are asked the question, "What plan do you want to choose," and answer: "Depends on the price"? You should never fall into a trap and present the price. As stated, the customer cannot answer the second question before answering the first. If you are tempted to get into the price at this stage, the answer will be, "I have to think about it." Of course there is need to think – if there has not been a decision as to which plan they want to choose, how will they decide if they are willing to pay the amount you are asking for?

Therefore, the answer to the customer at this stage should be, "Mr. Smith, we'll get to costs right away. It is only important that before we deal with financial matters you make a clean medical decision about your preferred program. With regard to costs – we will do our best so that the financial aspect will not be a problem. If the payment issue is a problem we will consider less expensive options."

The client may say at this point, "I prefer program C, which includes five permanent implants and four fillings." This simple answer seems to be a giant leap in terms of receiving the customer's consent, for the simple reason that now all he has left is to answer is the payment question. The dilemma over which treatment plan to undergo is already behind both of you.

In addition, this situation is optimal for you because the client will not have to hesitate with the receptionist or the practice manager about the treatment plan; he has already decided which one he prefers. All he and the receptionist will have to do now is discuss the price, discounts, payments, duration of the treatments, adjusting appointments to his needs, and so on.

Remember:
Customers tend to be suspicious of businesses and their intentions when it comes to money. This is even truer when it comes to dentistry, where there is a lot of uncertainty on the client's side, alongside very large price gaps between practices.

Therefore, when presenting alternatives to treatment programs, a great deal of attention is required to make sure that trust exists between the customers and the practice and that no suspicion is raised on the part of the clients regarding the practice's motives. A dental practice that is able to build trust between itself and its customers will win their hearts and their pockets; customers will not visit a practice that fails to develop a relationship based on trust.

A good method that can give you credit points and build trust is to give the customers the feeling that you care about their money too. For example, many dentists fail in this situation; when the customer asks them, "Doctor, what do you recommend?" they usually recommend the most expensive treatment plan (which in the majority of cases is truly the best plan). Oops – even if your recommendation is given to the customer with all your heart and without financial considerations, the customer is likely to think, "Hmm, I wonder why he is recommending the most expensive plan. Obviously he is just trying to make money off of me."

Therefore, you should begin to incorporate sensitivity and consideration for the customer's pocket. The answer to the question, "What do you recommend, Doctor?" could be, for example, "Mr. Smith, if you ask me, removable rehabilitation (prosthesis on implants) is an excellent option for you. It has many advantages, and mainly, it is much less expensive than the implant option alone. I have customers who have chosen this option and are very satisfied. If you want to upgrade to implants in the future, you can always do that."

By the way, if the customer has the budget needed for the expensive implant program, they will ask to hear more details about implants on their own. However, after hearing the explanation above, they will greatly appreciate the dentist's consideration for their pocket and will not feel that the expensive treatment is being pushed on them. Another example is to say to the customer, "Mr. Smith, you have two bridges; the bridge on the upper jaw is old and not in the best condition, but I would not replace it at the moment. Don't waste the money. You can use it for another two or three years. But I propose we replace the bridge on the lower jaw immediately." These messages are very important for building trust with the customer.

Chapter 12

Closing Treatment Plans

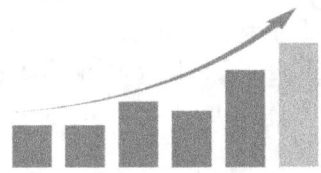

It is no accident that I chose to deal with closing the treatment plan only after discussing the practice's conduct toward its clients. The chance of selling a treatment plan depends entirely on the manner in which the practice operates up to this point. If clients experience unprofessional behavior and have a negative impression of the practice and its staff, there is no chance that they will agree to undergo treatment at this practice, even if they are sitting with a salesperson. However, appropriate conduct toward the clients in the preliminary stages "softens them up" and significantly increases the chance that they will decide to receive care at the practice – and to hell with the price!

However, even assuming that the practice's conduct was excellent up to closing the treatment plan, it is still true that big deals fall apart over small details. Therefore, make sure that the practice continues in the same manner and performs the closing stage efficiently.

I have come across quite a few practices whose conduct with clients was well executed and professional and then, at the decisive moment – the moment of closing the treatment plan – the team's conduct was amateur and lead to many lost transactions.

Why does this happen? Sales are not a simple matter. It is no coincidence that the sales profession is nicknamed the "art of selling." Receptionists at dental practices, who are involved in running the appointment book and maintaining continuous contact with the lab, do not always pay attention to sales. As if this were not enough, they do not always have the training required in order to sell treatment plans, especially when it comes to large sums. How many transactions can be lost due only to incorrect sales conduct? A great many!

A practice that I consulted and did very well in professional image and administrative conduct failed in the sales arena simply because it did not manage the sales chain properly. However, after the practice staff was trained in managing a correct and effective sales chain, the practice's sales tripled in comparison to the average annual sales. It's true that not every practice can double or triple its sales, but every practice can increase its percentage of closed treatment plans by at least 25%. This depends on the team's conduct throughout the sales chain. The more the links in the chain are effective and synchronized, the greater the chances of sales growth.

Before approaching clients in order to sell the treatment plan and build an effective sales chain it is desirable and worthwhile to synchronize the practice's sales approach, especially of those in charge of closing treatment plans. An incorrect sales approach is a sure recipe for lost deals, and I have encountered quite a few misguided approaches.

Here I will present the optimal sales approach for closing treatment plans. This approach is based on extensive experience in sales in general and in the field of selling treatment plans in dental practices in particular. Please note that the following sales approach is not experimental – it is implemented at a large number of dental practices around the world, and has been proven to increase sales significantly.

The Sales Approach at the Practice

One of the questions I ask the audience at my lectures to dentists and practice staff is, "Why do people care for their teeth?" The answers are usually predictable: aesthetics, toothaches, chewing quality, preventive treatment, etc. Then I ask the audience another question: "Wait a minute. If we take a random sample of ten people from the street and give them a dental exam, how many of them will need a treatment, even a small one?" The answer the audience gives is, "Everyone!" Then I ask the key question: "So if everyone needs treatment, where are they? Why aren't they coming in for a checkup?"

Well, the answer to this question is that the majority of clients go to a dental practice only when they have no choice. As long as they can postpone the treatments, they will. After all, they have more pressing and enjoyable things on which to spend their money. Therefore, the answer to the question, "Why do clients care for their teeth?" is, "Because they have no choice."

Why do I dwell on this seemingly minor matter? Because it is no small matter. The insight that clients take care of their teeth only when they have no choice changes the rules of the game when it comes to selling treatment plans. Any part of the practice team, and especially those involved in closing treatment plans, must internalize that if clients have reached the stage of calling the practice and asking for an appointment, they have already passed the procrastination stage and want care now! Actually, they don't just want care now – they need care now!

Furthermore, not only must they care for their teeth, but there is also a reasonable chance that they want to receive care from you. The fact that they chose to call your practice indicates that they must have received a good recommendation, that you are located close to their home, or some other reason. So assume that they want to receive care with you.

Why is this important? Because a major rule of sales is, "A prophecy fulfills itself." If you see potential clients as pests who just come to you for a quote and waste your time, then you will probably treat them as such, and so it will be. On the other hand, if you assume that they need care now and want to do this with you, then you will deal with them accordingly, and eventually they will become your clients.

Here's the bottom line: if clients came to your practice and are at the point of no choice, and came to you for a reason, then they must receive care with you. Moreover, if they decided not to receive care with you, something is probably wrong with one of the links in your sales chain. In order to reach a higher percentage of treatment plan sales in your practice, there are several important points that you and the practice staff should internalize.

A. **If there is no urgency; clients will not close the deal** – In order for clients to close the transaction they must understand that if they do not receive care now, the situation will only get worse: the pain will increase or they will eventually need more treatment that will cost much more. For example, from a normal filling the condition will worsen until they will need a root canal. If they do not internalize this, they will reject the treatment. As we have already said, they have many more important and fun things in which to invest their money. Therefore, the dentist, as well as the staff member who closes plans, should make the urgency of starting treatment clear to the client. For example, "Mr. Smith, I suggest a root canal treatment and treating the caries and inflammation so that, God forbid, you will not lose the tooth. If you lose the tooth you will need an implant and a crown that will cost you even more money." You can even use a little humor: "Mr. Smith, unfortunately teeth do not take care of themselves; it usually only gets worse."

B. **The client's right to bargain** – The two most common sentences I hear from practice staff are, "This is not a market!" and, "Why don't clients stop asking for a discount?" Ladies and gentlemen, the market – where there is bargaining – also has the highest percentage of deal-closing. So do you prefer that clients neither bargain nor close the deal, or that they do bargain and you close many treatment plans?

Consumer behavior has changed significantly in recent years, and one of the consequences is that clients go for discounts. Look at advertising: hardly any car, TV, or piece of furniture is sold without a discount. Therefore, if you want to try to "educate" your clients and run in the opposite direction from the consumer market, then the risk is entirely yours. By the way, I am repeatedly surprised by this; dentists are clients as well, and they buy their car and furniture as well as the equipment and materials for the practice only after receiving a discount. So why do they expect their clients not to ask for one?

It is worthwhile to understand a very important point about haggling over a price: haggling is one of the most effective tools for closing a deal (and not the opposite), and therefore you should not give it up. The following chapter will describe the manner of offering discounts without turning the practice into a flea market.

C. **Who closes the treatment plans at the practice – The dentist, practice manager, receptionists, or assistant?** The answer to this is very simple: the person who has the best chance of closing the most deals is the one who should close the treatment plans. Of course, the optimal situation is that the receptionists or the practice director closes the treatment plans, but there are practices where the receptionist or practice manager does not have spectacular sales skills.

If the receptionists have weak sales skills and the dentists are sales wizards, the dentists should take the most important role of all upon themselves – to enter into deals and work for the practice, while the receptionists will focus on negotiations, collection, and disbursements. It is unclear where the following strange idea came from, but unfortunately, it is very common in dental practices: The dentist does not deal with money. Clients ask the dentist how much the treatments cost, and the dentist, who has been working in the field for 25 years, replies, "I do not know the prices. The receptionists will sit down with you and discuss this." The dentist does not know how much implants cost? Is he detached from reality?

Clients know that they are in a private practice and it is clear to them that they are not in a place where free treatments are handed out, so there is no problem for the dentist to talk about the costs as well. Moreover, in practices where I recognized that the dentist had the highest chances of closing treatment plans, and after the dentist overcame the initial barrier of "A dentist does not deal with money," I was told that there was a significant increase in closing treatment plans.
In fact, if you think about it, there are a few good reasons why the dentist should close treatment plans:

1. It is more difficult for clients to bargain with the dentist than with the receptionists, precisely because of the awe and distance that I have already mentioned.

2. It is clear to clients that if they have any medical questions regarding the treatment plan, they can get a reliable and quick answer from the dentist.

3. As far as clients are concerned, the dentist can give the greatest discount – receptionists do not have enough authority in the matter.

4. In most cases, the dentist is more motivated to close the transaction (salary payments are coming up) than the receptionists are.

Indeed, quite a few dentists have taken the task of closing treatment plans upon themselves. They are not bad at all, and I have not heard of any clients complaining, "The dentist talks about money!" Despite all of the above, there is still an expectation that the practice manager or the receptionists perform the work of closing the treatment plans, because this leads to a waste of the dentists' precious time – and the assumption that they should devote their time to treatments rather than sales.

D. Exam day or examinations between treatments? – In most practices, clients who come in for an exam see the dentist between treatments. The dentist and practice staff are busy with treatments, so there is a reasonable chance that those who come for an exam will enter late or will not receive proper attention, and we already understand what the consequences here might be. Why, then, should the practice not allocate designated "exam hours" as needed, which will be kept on the books for this purpose alone? For example, Mondays from 5 PM to 7 PM and Wednesdays from 4 PM to 5 PM.

The main advantage of this is that the dentist and practice staff focus on closing business transactions during these hours. Everyone is more relaxed and set on closing plans. There are also fewer delays with appointments and you can make sure that the most suitable workers are present at these hours, etc. All of this may improve the carrying out and closing rates of treatment plans.

By the way, it is OK if a certain percentage of clients cannot make it during the specific hours designated for tests; the idea is that most of the exams will take place during these hours.

E. The price is not the main issue – The price is important to the clients, but other issues are more important to them, such as, *What are the chances of the treatment's success? Is the dentist a specialist in this field? What if the treatment fails?* Think about yourself as a client; when you buy products or services, is the price the only thing that matters to you? The answer is no. After all, you weigh the price with other parameters: quality, service, and so on. The clients in your practice are no different from you; they also think and act this way.

It is worth remembering that in the end, prices in different practices are quite similar. Specialists charge approximately the same prices, as do all public health practices, as well as most private practices. The differences, if any, range from 10 to 20%. This is not what will discourage clients.

Therefore, if those who close treatment plans are convinced that what interests clients is the price alone, they conduct themselves accordingly, thus making the price the main issue. Even if a client has a cheaper offer there is no reason for the closer to be defensive; on the contrary, a more expensive price may give you credit points (expensive = quality) and even raise doubts about the quality of a less expensive offer. When clients visit a Toyota dealership, do they say to the salesperson, "Listen, I have a cheaper offer from Subaru"? Definitely not. Although they both work, the Subaru is a Subaru, and the Toyota is a Toyota, just as Dr. Green is not Dr. Jones.

F. **Assist instead of convincing** – An effective sales approach, especially with skeptical clients, states that one should assist instead of convincing. When you try to convince clients to buy, you instinctively activate their defenses ("What are they trying to sell?"). On the other hand, when you try to help the clients make a purchase, you may actually activate the mechanisms of empathy ("Apparently they care for me").

So, how do you help clients? Imagine that a close friend is sitting in front of you. You will not try to convince them to undergo the treatment, but rather you will try to help them decide to perform the treatment in your practice because you are sure that this is best for them. You will not sit opposite them, but rather beside them, and you will not try to convince them that the price is good, but rather try to get them a good price. In fact, you will find yourself on their side rather than on the practice's side – "Let me talk to the dentist and the lab; I'll try to get you a discount." When the client feels that you are on their side, they are more open and willing to close a deal.

G. **Team Spirit** – Salespeople who believe in their product 100% – that there really is a justification for clients to pay more – will succeed in selling the most. Why? Because they project this to the clients. This equation works in the opposite direction as well: a salesperson who doubts the quality of the product and thinks that the clients have better alternatives will find it difficult to make sales. While closing a treatment plan you must firmly believe that if the clients undergo the treatment in another practice, even at a cheaper price, they will make a terrible mistake.

Therefore, it is important that whoever closes the treatment plans believes in the dentists and the product. The dentist and the practice owner (sometimes this is the same person) must produce team spirit in order for whoever closes the treatment plans to sell more. I know some receptionists who manage to sell many treatment plans for a certain dentist in the practice, but fail to close plans for another dentist at the same practice. Why? Because they cannot lie – they only know how to sell what they believe in.

Building a "Sales Chain" to Close Treatment Plans

In order to increase the chances of closing treatment plans there must be a correct and effective chain of sales. The sales chain is complete and effective cooperation between the dentists and the closers of the treatment plan (the receptionists or practice manager, in most cases). As we will find out later, an efficient and systematic sales chain is lacking in most practices. This makes it difficult to close deals.

In the vast majority of practices, the dentist comes to the receptionist with the treatment plan and says, "Please sit down with Mr. Smith and go over the plan and the costs." This is where the problems begin. The receptionists do not know the clients, what the preferred treatment plan is, what bothers the clients most, whether they are afraid of dental treatments, whether they have visited another practice and have another offer, where they have undergone treatment so far, who referred them to the practice, etc. This information is very important for the treatment plan and is usually known only by the dentist, who collected the information during the examination.

It is very important that you close the treatment plan with maximal information about the clients. This information can help direct the clients towards closing the deal quickly and efficiently. For example, if the closer of the treatment plan knows that the client previously received care in an inexpensive practice and was not satisfied with the quality of the treatment, he or she can tell the client, "I know that our prices are not cheap, but that's because we use the best quality materials, and the implants will be performed by a professional dentist with 17 years of experience. You've already learned that cheap treatments end up costing you dearly."

Or, if the client indicated to the dentist that they have both implants and a removable prosthesis, and that they are satisfied with the implants but will not hear of another removable prosthesis, the closer must know not to insist on a removable prosthesis, and secondly, that the client is familiar with dental implants both medically and financially.

The client's transition from the exam stage to the sales stage at the receptionist's desk has to be smooth and perfect, just as a runner in a relay race has to transfer the baton to the runner behind them without dropping it or slowing down.

There are two options for creating an effective sales chain between the dentist and the closer.

The first option is for the receptionist to be present in the treatment room throughout the examination. During the exam they will be able to collect all the information required in order to close the deal. In addition, they will be able to interact with the clients before talking to them about costs, making it is easier for all of them. This option is effective and can be implemented when you plan examination slots (special hours for checkups, remember?) and then backup the receptionists' station. This is optimal when there is a full-time practice manager who can be present at the examinations without affecting the receptionists' station.

In a large practice that I consulted for, I served as a closer among other roles. I enjoyed every moment. I would arrive on the day of examinations and be in close contact with the senior dentist in the treatment room during checkups. The information I gathered about the clients and their needs contributed greatly to closing the treatment plans, which I did almost without a problem. It is difficult to imagine what the percentage of closed deals would have been had I not had this information.

Most practices, especially small and medium-sized ones, cannot implement this option because of an objective lack of a manager or receptionists to accompany the dentist for any length of time during the exam. Therefore, such practices can adopt the second option: a minimized sale chain that is also very effective.

The second option is carried out as follows: The dentist performs the initial exam with the assistant only, and when the stage of presenting alternatives for the client's treatment plans arrives, they call the receptionist into the treatment room and perform a "hot transfer." The dentist presents the receptionist to the client and provides a brief overview: "Ms. Green was referred to us by Samson. She received an offer from another practice that included X, Y, and Z. I offered her alternatives S and T, and she preferred to carry out the T program. She has a normal cavity that needs treatment very urgently so that, God forbid, it does not turn into a root canal, and a wisdom tooth that must be extracted immediately because it is pushing on the tooth next to it." At the end of the review, have the dentist add, "Please give her a good price and a payment plan."

There are several advantages in transferring clients to the receptionist in such a way:
A. The treatment plan closer now has important information that can be used for closing the transaction.

B. The dentist, client, and receptionist know which program the client prefers, which greatly reduces the number of medical questions that the client will need to ask the receptionist. What remains now is to discuss the price.

C. The receptionist does not have to start from scratch, since an interaction has already been created. ("You're related to Samson? He's a great fellow. Say 'hi' to him for me!")

D. The dentist created a sense of urgency for starting the treatment. The urgency is clear to both the client and the receptionist.

E. The dentist sparks empathy and a good feeling in the client when he says, "Give her a discount," which the receptionist can take advantage of during the sale.

In order to remove any doubt, the most important point in the sales chain is that clients should be transferred from the dentist to the receptionist only under the following circumstances:

1. The customer has decided which treatment they prefer.

2. The dentist has created a sense of urgency (if there is cause for this, of course) about starting with something small such as a regular filling or extraction.

3. The dentist instructs the receptionist, "Give them a good price."

The Location of Closing the Treatment Plan

Before I specify what to do and what not to do in order to close a treatment plan in the best way, I will address an important point that may affect the entire interaction: the location of closing the treatment plan. Most practices do not arrange the building correctly, and the critical phase of the sale is performed at the reception station. Yes, at the reception station – where there is no privacy, where clients do not feel comfortable asking for a discount or a more extensive payment plan (someone is standing right next to them), and in the meantime, the receptionist is also forced to answer the phone and set up appointments for other clients who are in a hurry. How are they supposed to discuss a complex treatment plan with Mr. Smith and how is he supposed to make a decision that will cost possibly thousands of dollars? It is very important that there be privacy and that all the receptionist's attention be directed at him. Mr. Smith has questions and concerns, wants explanations or to ask for a discount, or an option for spreading out the payments, etc. If Mr. Smith does not receive the receptionist's full attention, he will remain with unanswered questions and unable to make a decision about closing the deal. Even the interruptions and noise around – phones, etc. – can impair the receptionist's concentration and reduce the chances of closing the deal.

The optimal situation is to make the sale in a separate and closed room that emits professionalism. The table should be organized, training certificates should be placed in front of the client, and nothing should interfere with the receptionist and Mr. Smith's discussion about the treatment plan. If you have a room of this type, use it. However, such a room does not exists in most practices and therefore an alternative is to find a corner of the reception station to allow for some privacy in order to hold the sales pitch. The client should sit rather than stand – they have not heard the price yet – and a barrier must be created between the client and the rest of the receptionist's activities.

In some cases, it is even possible to give the sales pitch in the treatment room, when there is no other patient in the room. You can designate a small sitting area where the dentist or receptionist can explain the treatment plan. Despite the inconvenience, this is better than a noisy and busy office.

The Six Stages of Closing a Treatment Plan

The more the previous stages, and especially the sales stage, proceed correctly and professionally, the easier it will be for receptionist to close the treatment plan. In many cases, when the client knows the approximate price range and expresses confidence in the dentists and even shows positive signs of closure such as, "My daughter is getting married in two months; can I finish the treatment by then?", all that remains is for the receptionist to set up a quick appointment and present the costs and payment arrangements.

However, with a more complex treatment plan and higher costs, especially when it comes to transplants and rehabilitations, a more orderly sales pitch is required. It is best that the closer study all the steps thoroughly and know exactly what to do at each stage. Knowing what to do at any given stage will prepare them for questions or any resistance on the part of the clients, give them confidence, and increase the percentage of closed treatment plans.

The sale of the treatment plan is divided into six steps.
1. Creating closeness
2. Presenting the treatment plan
3. Displaying the price
4. Handling objections and negotiating
5. Closing the plan
6. Monitoring treatment plans that have not been closed

Step One – Creating Closeness

Every sale, wherever it may be, begins with the creation of closeness. Sales and marketing experts call this the "softening phase." The better it is, the easier it will become. Sales experts devote most of their time to creating closeness because the sales pitch, in many cases, begins and ends there. If trust and sympathy are created between the seller and buyer, all other matters are easily resolved. The opposite is true as well.

Therefore, it is not advisable to seat a client down and immediately talk to them about the costs, but rather to try to develop a relationship with them in the following style: "I understand that Samson referred you to us. How is he? Give him my best and thank him for sending us so many clients."

Finding a common denominator with the client also creates closeness and it is worthwhile to use this technique. For example, "Is your son in the same kindergarten as Lucy? I am very pleased with the kindergarten teachers," etc.

Step Two – Presenting the Treatment Plan

Before running to show the client the treatment plan, you must set the groundwork and make sure that they know and understand all of the practice's competitive advantages, and therefore, immediately after the small talk and before the treatment plan is presented, you must "review" the practice. For the purpose of the review, a presentation or brochure can be used. It should not be longer than one minute but these messages are very important in order to differentiate yourself from other competitors that the client has visited or may visit down the road. It should go something like this:

"Mr. Smith, before we move on to the treatment plan, I want to tell you a little about our practice. The practice was established 21 years ago by Dr. Jones, and she is the medical director. The practice provides all the treatments under one roof. Dentists from various fields are employed here, and every dentist performs the treatments in his or her area of expertise. Dr. Jones performs root canal treatments; Dr. Kumar performs orthodontic treatment; (etc.). Your treatments will be performed by three dentists: Dr. Gold, an expert in oral and maxillofacial surgery from a well-known hospital, will perform the dental implant treatment. Dr. Jones will perform the root canal treatments and Dr. Green will perform the oral rehabilitation stage. It's important to note that we work at the highest standards in terms of materials and lab work, and since dental care is not particularly pleasant, we try to give the best and most empathetic service to our clients. I'll accompany you personally throughout your treatments here at the practice. Feel free to read about us in more detail in the practice brochure, which I will give you along with the treatment plan. Do you have any questions? Great, then let's continue with the treatment plan."

After this introduction, you should pay attention to the following important detail: the client must not be handed the treatment plan before receiving an explanation. Why? Because clients will immediately begin to wonder about the cost and be preoccupied with the price from that moment on and where the money will come from. Therefore, at this first stage it is recommended that the treatment plan stay in the receptionist's hands.

The receptionist will present the client's preferred treatment plan as previously indicated to them by the dentist. The receptionist will review the overall plan with the client: how long it may take, how many visits are expected, whether lab work is necessary, and most importantly create a sense of urgency about starting treatment. Here is an example for presenting the program:

"Mr. Smith, Dr. Jones's treatment plan, which was your top choice, includes three transplants, three structures and crowns, two fillings, and the extraction of a wisdom tooth. We estimate that the entire plan will take six months. In addition, we will need to take measurements and send them to the lab. You will need about 12 visits. I want to emphasize, as Dr. Jones pointed out, that the extraction of the wisdom tooth and two fillings should begin immediately so that you will not need painful and expensive root canal treatments."

The marketing logic is simple: the client hears the price of the treatment process only after they know how many visits the program entails, how long the program might last, and that it includes lab work; they will understand what they are paying for and what the price entails. If the client hears the price before hearing about the process, the first question will be, "Why is it so expensive?"

After a brief breakdown of the process, the receptionist should wait a little before arriving at the costs, in order to see that the client understands and agrees with the treatment plan. Present the price only after the client asks, "How much does it cost?" This means that we can move on to the next stage only after the client has understood the treatment plan.

Step Three – Displaying the Price

As noted in the sales approach at the beginning of the chapter, it is advisable to give the clients a discount. It is best for the receptionist to be one to initiate the discount and present it along with the price. There are a number of reasons for this. First, about 90% of clients request and receive a discount in any case. Second, giving an initial discount places the client in the negotiation arena and creates an atmosphere of closing the transaction. Third, granting a discount gives the receptionist credit points with the clients ("They like me"). Besides, remember the dentist asking the receptionist to give the client a good deal?

In addition, the practice wants the client to leave with the feeling that they received a discount. Imagine what goes through the mind of loyal clients who have been coming to the practice along with their entire family, and pay a full price without a discount. There is no better way to show clients that their loyalty is appreciated than to give them a discount and allow them to make convenient payments.

The discount does not harm profitability; it is advisable to add 10-15% to the usual prices so that there will both be room for a discount and you will remain profitable – exactly as all commercial companies do. Those who think that you start at the price you want to accept and close deals with the clients without a discount, especially when it comes to large treatment plans, apparently do not understand the rules of the current market; they will have a life of difficult negotiations and low closing levels. Giving clients a discount is one of the most effective tools for closing a deal. However, this step should be done wisely and carefully.

Here are six tips on how to use the discount as an effective tool for closing a deal.

1. **If you do not initiate, you will end up following rather than leading** – Providing a discount proactively may reduce the client's desire (and need) to ask for a discount and bargain for the price. If the client asks for another discount, the receptionist can always argue that "the price is after a discount" and you may be able to settle for more payments in order to close the deal. Hence, when the receptionist initiates the discount, they lead the negotiation rather than follow the client's demands.

   For example, the receptionist presents Mr. Smith with the regular price of $12,890. After a discount the price is $11,800 (a discount of $1,090); they communicate to him that even if he gets another discount, it will not be in big leaps because they have already determined the level of the discount. On the other hand, if the receptionist does not initiate the discount, the client may demand a discount of $4,000. With a starting point on the client's side, it will be difficult for the receptionist to cope.

2. **The discount should be stated in sums rather than percentages** – Especially when it comes to large sums, stating the discount as a percentage is good for the client but bad for you. To client, who gets a 10% discount, it seems small (after all, yesterday they bought cloths for 50% off and electrical appliances for 35% off). Therefore, specify the discount in terms of the amount of money it comes out to (for example, $860). The discount will sound a lot more significant to the client this way. In addition, if the discount is specified as a percentage, the client may request another discount, also as a percentage – "Give me another 10%." This is a small percentage to them but a lot of money for you.

3. **Do not be cheap but do not exaggerate** – A tiny discount will not tempt the client to perform the treatment. A huge discount may be seen as unreliable or encourage the client to ask for another large discount. My recommendation for the discount in dental practices is as follows: 8% off the initial price, 4% after the client asks for another discount, and 1% to round the price off: a total of 13%. Again, this discount is after being added to the initial price, so even if you use all of it you will still make a profit and get your desired price. Calculating the percentages should be done using a calculator and presented to the client as a specific amount.

4. **Let the client have the final word** – The receptionist should be prepared for the fact that in many cases, in addition to the discount they gave, the client will request an additional discount. Hence, the receptionist must leave more room for maneuvering with the price. In fact, the optimal situation is that the client indicates the price they want to pay and close the deal themselves. Negotiation experts know how to address this situation; for example, they will deliberately offer the client a price of $1,090 after discount, knowing that the client will close the deal themselves when they ask to lower it to $1,000.

5. **Does the client want another discount? Let them fight for it.** Clients who ask for a certain discount and receive a quick positive answer will probably not close the deal. Why? Because they think to themselves (and rightly so), "If I had asked for a larger discount I might have received it." Even if the client's request is worthwhile and profitable for the practice, it is important to say 'No' at first and agree only after efforts on the part of the client. A discount received easily is not appreciated; however, if the client received the discount after fighting for it, they feel victorious. And what is better than clients who feel they have won? Another point in this context is that the receptionist cannot give the extra discount (over the first 8%) on their own, in order not to undermine their credibility. "If they could give a bigger discount, why did they not do this in the first place?" the clients will think. Therefore, confirmation of the additional discount should be received from the dentist or the practice owner. Acting skills can definitely be useful at this stage.

6. **Reliability** – Discounts do not gain greater credibility with consumers. Moreover, they are perceived as a marketing tactic to promote sales rather than as concern for consumers' welfare. Therefore, the receptionist should take a few steps to add a measure of reliability to the discount.

   First, it is recommended to add a good and satisfactory reason for the discount, for example, "As loyal clients of ours, you deserve..." or, "Since you were referred to our practice by Samson...." Second, using exact prices conveys the message that the price and discount were reached with seriousness and thoroughness – "The price is $1,240 before the discount and $1,120 after the discount" – as opposed to round prices like $2,000. By the way, prices such as 99 lost their psychological effectiveness long ago.

Presenting the price to the client should be as follows: "Mr. Smith, the total price of your treatment plan is 14,860 [a non-rounded price], but as a long-time client of the practice [reason for the discount] you deserve a discount of 960 [specifying the discount in money and not in percentages]. The price after discount is 13,900. Additionally, I can spread out your payments."

A well-known rule of every sales expert is that after telling the client the price, remain silent and wait to hear his or her reaction. There are two reasons for this: First, those who speak after the price is mentioned apparently do not believe in the price they noted (a lack of confidence and). Second, you need to get the client's response to the price in order to design the most effective response.

Step Four – Handling Objections

It is reasonable to assume that after the client hears the price they will express objections. This is true mainly with respect to medium- and large-scale plans, which cost thousands of dollars and more, and constitute a difficult financial burden for the client. Clients raise objections to a proposal for several reasons: **A.** This is a tactic to improve buying conditions, or in other words, "I won't pay this amount; you will give me a discount." **B.** The client expresses a gap between expectations and what was offered – dental treatments are always more expensive than expected. **C.** Perhaps the main reason: this is an economic risk for the client, who is afraid of making a bad purchasing decision and therefore needs reassurance that they are making the right decision.

The receptionist should be prepared, and have an answer for any possible resistance. The receptionist's preparation and having a correct answer to all types of resistance gives them an advantage and reduces the chance of making mistakes at this critical stage. Before I specify what types of objections the clients may raise and how the receptionist must respond to any resistance, it is worth clarifying three key issues related to effectively addressing objections.

Objections are actually good – Objections are actually a positive signal, indicating that the client is interested in making the purchase. Confused? Here's the logic: if the client has no interest in the purchase, they would be indifferent and therefore not raise objections. Someone living on the North Pole will not object to the price of a freezer being offered to him since he had no interest in the product anyway. Therefore, when the client expresses resistance, you should see it as a positive sign – they want to receive care at your practice, and that already constitutes 80% of the sale. Now they just need reassurance for this decision.

Always, always agree with client's resistance – the first step in handling any resistance is to agree with the client. If they say "Expensive!" and the receptionist answers, "It's not expensive," or, "Expensive compared to what?" they will go down an argumentative road rather than a smooth one. The client is busy proving that they are right (that the price is expensive) and insulted that you disagree with them. However, if the receptionist agrees with their claim and answers, "Yes, it is a large investment – dental treatments are not cheap," they feel agreed with. Please make sure to use the term 'investment' rather than 'expense.' Once the client has been softened, other messages can easily be communicated. By the way, it really does not matter whether or not the client's resistance is justified. The important thing at the first stage is to soften them and not create a dispute.

When the clients ask questions, what do they mean? An integral part of closing plans is dealing with medical questions from patients: What implant do you use? What is a sinus lift? And so on, and so forth.

It is precisely in this area that many of the practice's staff fail and begin to explain everything they know about dentistry. The result? Confused clients are full of information but cannot make a purchase decision and want to go home to process the great deal of information they received.

What is the answer when the client asks, "Which implants do you use?" Whoever answers by stating the brand names (*Mis*, *Alpha*, *Bio*, etc.) probably did not understand the question. Do you really think that the clients are interested in the brand name of the implants? Moreover, if you tell them the brand name, what are they supposed to do with it?

Ladies and gentlemen, you should understand and internalize this: clients ask questions not because they want to study dentistry but because they are afraid and want to reduce uncertainty. Will the answer "We use *Mis* implants" help reduce their uncertainty? Absolutely not. On the contrary! They will ask, "Are *Mis* implants good? What is the difference between the various brands of implants?" And so on.

Therefore, the correct answer to the question of which implants you use is, "Mr. Smith, don't worry; we use the best implants. Dr. Kumar has performed thousands of implants with a success rate of about 96%. You're in the best hands." That's what the clients want to hear: that they are in good hands. After all, they do not know what the dentist is doing in their mouth, and therefore, what is most important is that they trust the dentist. Once they trust the dentist, they trust them to use the implants in the best and most suitable way for the case.

Beyond this, a basic rule of sales says that the more information you give the clients the more you keep them away from buying. There are two reasons for this: first, you broadcast insecurity and second, you give them information to think about. So, you have to answer the clients but it is important that the answers be in broad terms, and that the messages be reassuring and reduce uncertainty, without going into detail about which implants you use and how the bone is implanted during the sinus lift.

I'll end with a little story that illustrates the point. A few years ago, I had a nice client who loved surgery very much. He loved surgery so much that he used to travel abroad and give lectures as a representative of an implant company. Assessing his practice, I found that the closing percentages were low. When I observed an examination he was conducting, I understood why – he was lecturing clients who came for an examination about surgery: how implants are placed, where you place the implant, which type of implant is suitable for this case, etc. The result? Clients would go home to think about it.

I explained the side effects of overwhelming clients with information, and did another thing: we limited his tests to 20 minutes. The receptionists would give him a sign after fifteen minutes that only 5 minutes were left. He was disciplined and indeed stuck to the schedule and stopped elaborating. Additionally, I gave him a set of (soothing) messages that he was to pass on to the clients during the test. The result? His closing rates increased significantly, as did the practice's sales.

The Tactic of Handling Objections

Increasing closeness leads to fewer objections – the more the receptionist manages to create a relationship with the client in the first stages of the sale, the fewer objections they will have. If the receptionist is able to make the client like them and see them as reliable and trustworthy, it is likely that they will have fewer reservations, and if they do have them, they will share them with the receptionist, which is a huge step on the way to closing the deal. By the way, it is worthwhile to learn from the Japanese: before they talk business, they take clients out for a good meal or a game of golf.

Reduce Objections – If it were not so important, I would not repeat this advice again. Want fewer objections? Get a "Yes!" from the client for a certain treatment and only then talk about the price. "Mr. Smith, before we approach the price, I wanted to make sure that you have decided that you want the dental implants and not the dentures." If the client answers "Yes," the next step will be easier for the client as well as for the receptionist, since all that is left is to reach an agreement on the price. If there is no "Yes" to the plan, there will be many objections since the client is not sure about what they want to do.

A few more tips:

A. Listen carefully; sometimes objections arise from lack of communication.

B. Talk about the difference rather than the total amount: "It is worth settling for a lesser treatment when the difference is only $1,200?"

C. Insist on a fair comparison: for example, "Mr. Smith, they are a public dental practice (with everything that entails), and we are a private practice. It's like comparing apples to oranges."

D. Even if the client uses tricks, do not take it personally – play the game.

Effectively Handling Objections and Negotiations

No matter how you look at it, after you show the client the price of a plan plus the discount – and of course remain proactively silent to get their response to the proposal – there are only four ways for them to respond to your proposal:

Let's go from easy to difficult:

1. "Okay, when can we start?"
2. "That's expensive! Give me another discount."
3. "Wow, that's expensive!"
4. "Let me think about it."

It is best for the receptionist to be prepared for every response, to understand what the client means with every response, and what the best reaction is to any response from the client. Let's go over all four common client responses and how to address each one.

"Okay, when can we start?" This is the dream scenario for closing a plan. Sometimes dreams come true; it happens mainly when the client has no idea about prices – they received a very warm recommendation about the dentist and practice. And, yes, there are those who do not ask for another discount. What the receptionist should do at this point is shake the client's hand and say, "Good luck to all of us!" In addition, the receptionist must schedule an appointment in the near future and ask for an advance of a certain percentage of the total treatment plan.

Why should we do this? Because this is a sensitive time, in which the client may change their mind. In professional jargon, this phenomenon is called cognitive dissonance – after people make a decision they often wonder, "Did I make the right decision?" Once they feel insecure about their decision they may reverse it, or at least reject it: "You know what, let me think about it a little more." The handshake and a financial advance locks them down and lets them know that there is no way back, which makes it difficult for them to think about the possibility of going back on the decision or rejecting it.

"That's expensive! Give me another discount." – This is a common form of resistance that we need to know how to handle correctly. First, it is important to understand what the client means when they say this. Usually they mean that they want the treatment being offered to them, here and now. They just want a discount on the price, which is very legitimate. In fact, when the client expresses this objection, about 80% of the sale had already been completed. This situation is excellent for closing the treatment plan – it is easier to get to the desired price than to convince the client that this is the right place to undergo the treatment. Therefore, the closer of the treatment plan should be very happy when they encounter this type of resistance.

How do you react to such resistance? As I suggested at the price presentation stage, the client has already received a discount on the initial price. If the receptionist gives another discount, they may be perceived as unreliable. Therefore, the receptionist's initial answer should be, "It's true that this is no small investment. This is made up of X dental implants, Y crowns, and (so on). The price I'm giving you is after a discount, but I can check about another discount for you."

At this second stage, the receptionist should ask the client for something in exchange for the additional discount: "Mr. Smith, how much cash can you pay out of the total amount?" There is a rule in negotiations according to which if you give something up, the other side has to give up something too; just like we interact with children: "If you want me to buy you the robot, you have to do your chores."

After the client expresses their willingness to pay even 20% of the total amount in cash, the receptionist should use another factor to give an additional discount: the dentist or the practice owner. As I mentioned, at this point the receptionist is on the client's side and fighting for them to receive another discount (and perform the treatments here). Acting skills are required: the receptionist will go to the dentist or owner and come back with another discount to close the deal: "Mr. Smith, the dentist is in a good mood today – I got you another discount."

"**Wow, that's expensive!**" – This is a very common, difficult, and complex type of resistance compared to the previous type. This is because the clients do not say they want another discount, and therefore it is impossible to know whether they even want to close a deal. However, it is worth remembering that this is a positive objection – usually clients do not say "expensive" about something in which they have no interest. Another thing worth remembering is that resistance is reserved for negotiation experts. Clients who raise such an objection will say that the price is expensive no matter what you say. Why? Because they want to put you on the defensive for the price negotiations. By the way, it's rare to meet clients who say, "Wow, what a cheap price. In another practice they asked for a lot more!"

Another reason customers might say that the price is high is the objective fact that they did not expect such a price, and they are just thinking, *Where will I get that amount?* However, as time passes the customer will begin to digest the price and realize that these are the prices of dental treatments – "My brother had dental implant treatment for $45,000" they will recall. In any case, we should not think that when customers say "expensive" they mean that they have had a cheaper offer. Treatment plans are often not the same.

The approach to this resistance includes three steps, to be performed in the following order:

1. **Agree with the client** – Agreement reduces resistance, as opposed to a disagreement, which could lead to debate and intensify opposition. Therefore, after the client says, *"Wow, expensive,"* the receptionist should look at them empathically and agree, *"You are right, Mr. Smith, this is not a small investment,"* and add the statement: *"Dental care is not a cheap matter."*

2. **Strengthen the client's choice** – At the second stage of handling resistance, the receptionist should convey two messages to the client: First, the treatment plan is not cheap because it includes many treatments, expensive materials, quality lab work, and so on. Clients should not think that the treatment plan is expensive because the practice is making a lot of money at their expense. Second, they are making the right decision despite the high price.

   It should go like this: "Mr. Smith, your treatment plan is complex and includes a lot of work. You have to undergo six transplants, a sinus lift, and a lot of lab work; it's a long process of about one year from the beginning of treatment. In the end it will pay off – you will not have to use the dentures that bother you today, and you will be able to eat all the food you can only dream of now."

3. **Another discount as a condition for closing the deal** – At this stage it is advisable to sweeten the deal and offer another discount, as a condition for closing the deal. "Mr. Smith, as I mentioned, the price is after a discount; but because it is a great plan, and since you're a loyal client, I'll do anything to get you another discount and a convenient payment plan, so that you can start treatment right away." **The receptionist should** remain silent **and wait for the client to ask,** "How much of a discount?" **Pay attention to the following: the client has now moved to a different type of resistance, which is easier to deal with – they ask for another discount. All that remains is for the receptionist to switch to the easier kind of resistance, from the previous section.

"Let me think about it" – This is undoubtedly the most difficult and complex form of resistance: what do the clients mean when they say they want to think about it? Probably to think about what has been offered because they cannot make a decision here and now. Few of us can make a quick decision about a transaction worth thousands of dollars. We have to digest it, consult with our partner, bank manager, etc. Therefore, it is wrong to view this resistance as a negative evasion or lack of interest. As you probably know, many clients have thought about the plan and came back to undergo it.

As noted, you should always agree with the client's objections. The same applies to this resistance, therefore the best answer to this objection would be, "No problem, Mr. Smith; take your time and think about it."

However, here it is worthwhile to initiate another **silence**. When the receptionist is quiet, the client feels the need to say something; most likely, they will reveal what it is that they want to think about. In addition, legitimizing the client's wish to take the time and think conveys that the practice is confident about the price and that they are not afraid of clients thinking about the offer. Do not say, "What do you want to think about?" or, "What is there to think about?" and so on. This shows a lack of confidence on the part of the practice, as well as a lack of respect for clients and their wishes.

There is a small addition to this stage – after all, we do not give up and release the clients too quickly. As we recall, we agreed that the treatment plan would include at least one or two treatments that are "very urgent." Here is the place to "release" the clients to think, but "catch" them simultaneously. This starts with the small and urgent part of the program. If the client starts part of the treatment and is satisfied with it, it is reasonable to assume that they will also want to continue with the treatment.

"Mr. Smith, no problem; I understand that you have to think about a financial expense of $28,000 and consult with your family. I just wanted to emphasize that there is a tooth extraction and a regular filling that Dr. Jones noted which, regardless of the plan, must be dealt with before the matter gets worse. The cost for these two treatments is a total of $640, so I will be happy to set up an urgent appointment so you can get it over with. As for the rest of the program, take your time; in the meantime I'll see if it's possible to accommodate you a little more with the price and the payment plan."

The name of the game at the closing point is timing. It's like a first kiss: if you try too soon, you'll be slapped. If you try too late, they'll think that something is wrong. If so, what is the right time to close the deal? You have to listen to the client in order to know. The receptionist should pay attention to the client's purchase signals. When the client asks, "How long will it take to complete the treatment?" or, "Is it possible to do morning appointments?" they are signaling that the other things are already agreed upon and it is possible to move on in order to close the deal.

The receptionist will address 'closing questions' to clients who signal the closing of the transaction with, "Ms. Green, do you want me to make an appointment for next week so you can finish this?" If the client responds in the affirmative – congratulations! If they agree to the appointment, they expressed consent and actually closed the deal themselves.

Step Five – Closing the Treatment Plan

The closing stage of the sale process is once again similar to the first kiss: the secret is timing. If you try too soon, you might be slapped. If you try too late, you may become irrelevant. Here are five tips for closing the treatment plan correctly.

1. If you don't remain quiet, how will you close the deal?

Research shows that the most common cause of failure at the closing stage is fear. Sales people are so afraid that the client will say 'no' that they continue to talk and talk, assuming that this will close the deal. However, extra talk during the closing phase causes the opposite reaction: disruption of momentum and raising doubts, all of which diminishes the chance of closing a deal. Moreover, extra talk creates a sense of over-selling and a lack of confidence on the part of the deal closer, and makes them look like someone who does not believe in the price and quality of the treatment. Therefore, at the closing stage, the closer must be assertive and pass the ball to the client's court, using deliberate silences. You'll be surprised – if you stay quiet for a moment, the clients may ask you, "Where do I sign?"

2. Use the "Fuse Test"

In order for the client to agree to close the treatment plan, they need to agree to several things: the treatment plan, price, payment terms, and more. However, often, the treatment plan closer leads the client to the closing stage before the client has agreed to all of these. In such a situation, the prospect of closing the deal is slim. Before you try to close the deal, it is worth using the fuse method used by electricians: testing each fuse separately to see what is blocking electricity from passing through the circuit. For example, "So let's sum things up, Mr. Smith. I understand you've decided on the implant program and not on dentures – great. I also understand that the price is acceptable to you – great," and so on. If you encounter a 'burnt fuse,' you have to address it individually and only then move on towards closing the deal. By the way, it is worth starting with the agreed-upon issues. The more the clients say, "Yes," at the beginning, the more likely it is that the closing of the transaction will be successful.

3. Offer another discount as a condition of closing the deal

Using discounts is one of the most effective methods of closing a deal, but in order for it to succeed, it is best to leave an adequate margin in the quote in case the client asks for a discount in addition to the one they already received. In order not to compromise the treatment plan closer's reliability, it is recommended that you approve the additional discount with the practice owner (usually the dentist). It is important that the closer does not contact the owner of the practice for another discount before receiving a commitment from the client for closing the transaction, and even a concession on their part, obtained gently, in a particular area. For example, "Mr. Smith, with your permission, I will try to convince the dentist to give you another discount in addition to the one I gave you. Can you pay 40% of the price in cash in return? I'm sure this will help us get another discount."

4. Don't Hesitate

Hesitation on the part of closer, at the closing stage, may lead to hesitation on the client's part, and vice versa: if the closer sends the clients a confident message about the transaction being carried out, it is reasonable to assume that it will indeed take place. At the closing stage, do not ask the client hesitantly, "What did you decide?" Instead, ask confidently, "Is it alright for you to undergo the treatment in the evenings, or do you prefer mornings?" Either way, you'll win as they will either answer mornings/evenings and thereby close the deal themselves, or will say that they have not decided yet and voice an objection – in this case, you can handle the objection and close the deal. This method is only relevant when the closer feels that the client is ready to close and all that is required is another small push.

5. Pay Attention to the Client's Signals

The client's body language and the questions they ask can give you a clear idea about whether they are ready to close or whether you have more work to do. Clients who ask, "How long after treatment is it possible return to work?" give you a green light to set up appointments and arrange payment. On the other hand, if the client sits opposite you with their hands and legs crossed and their body leaning back, you have quite a bit of persuading to do.

Step Six – Follow-Up: Monitoring a Treatment Plan that Has Not Been Closed

In observations I have conducted at many practices, I found that one of the major failures occurs during the follow-up of plans that have not been closed. "Why should we chase the clients? They said they would call us," the receptionists answer when asked about follow-up, thus exempting themselves from this process. This isn't supposed to comfort you, but this failure is characteristic of almost every salesperson out there.

Monitoring a treatment plan that has not been closed is as important as conducting negotiations with the clients when they are in the practice. Practices lose a lot of money because of not conducting the follow up stage properly, or worse, not performing this stage at all. I have proved this to a large number of practices. After they began to perform the follow-up phase correctly, they discovered to their surprise that clients could be returned to the practice and sales turnover increased significantly and quite easily.

The main problem is that many receptionists see this stage as their being a nuisance if they contact the client after they went home and promised to call. However, that's a mistake! The clients came to the practice voluntarily – you did not kidnap them off the street. You entertained them, the dentist devoted time to a checkup, and you made them an offer, therefore it is your right – your obligation, even – to call and find out what they think of the offer. Of course, if they say they do not want you to call them anymore, or that they have begun treatment at another practice, you should respect this and wish them success.

Another reason that receptionists do not thoroughly carry out this stage of my method is lack of time. True, they're busy sending out reminders to tomorrow's clients, making sure the lab work has arrived, etc. Nevertheless, ladies and gentlemen, should we really ignore the follow-up? After all, one of the most important things is the introduction of new patients – and therefore income – to the practice.

Basic and methodical follow up is one of the largest growth and income engines for the practice because clients, who go home to think about the proposal, are simply postponing their purchase decision. This does not mean they do not want to take care of their teeth; after all, they visited the practice for a reason. They just need some time to conduct all sorts of calculations, and not only financial ones, before they make a decision.

A study of consumer behavior has found that 73% of clients make large and complex purchases after about four rejections! The same study also showed that most sales people give up after the first or second refusal by the client. Only a small number of salespeople manage to sell to many clients. Therefore, the follow up is intended for direct contact with the clients who usually check out more offers, to make sure that when they decide, your practice will be high on their list.

By the way, clients often ask to "think about it" because they want to check out other alternatives, but in practice, they do not always have the time and energy to do so. So, a few days after visiting you at the practice, they probably still have not found the time to make appointments at other practices, and assuming that the dental problem did not resolved itself, this is the best time to bait them to start treatment with you.

In one of the workshops I conducted for the staff of a small dental practice, I asked for a list of clients who had been offered a treatment plan in the past two weeks and had not yet closed. We decided to do a simulation and call a random client to demonstrate how to conduct the follow-up. I asked the receptionist to call a certain client from the list, ask him how he was, and say, "Well, when should we schedule an appointment for?" The receptionist called the client and turned on the loudspeaker so that the whole team could hear the call. The selected client was a taxi driver on the job, who answered exactly according to the scheme I had presented to the practice a few minutes earlier: "I wanted to go to another practice for another offer but I can't find the time."

It is very possible that if the receptionist had not called this client, time would have passed, he would have found the time to go to a practice his friend recommended and closed a treatment plan there. It is worth clarifying another point, in order to clear up any doubt – receptionists who systematically monitor clients not only do not come across as nagging, but the opposite; the receptionist is viewed as a professional who does their job faithfully and shows that they really care about the clients. On the other hand, a practice that does not contact clients who visited them may be perceived as too overloaded or too hectic, which will lead clients not to want to receive care there anyway.

Ways to Carry Out the Follow-Up

I've come across all kinds of follow-up methods for plans that have not been closed: lists on the computer, Excel tables, folders with printed pages, etc. There is no preferable method. On a tactical level, everyone should use the method that is most convenient for him or her. However, on a strategic level, in order for the monitoring to be effective, it must be based on a number of principles that are important to keep in mind. The process I will present here refers to the (good) old method of a binder with printed pages, but as mentioned above, the process can also be performed using Excel sheets on your computer. Here is the process.

A. **Dedicated binder for treatment plans** – Every treatment plan proposal should be printed out in three copies: one for the client, a second to the client's medical file, and another for the treatment plan folder, which will hold all the proposals given by the practice. The advantage lays in the fact that important data is easily accessible to the receptionists: the date of the proposal, which dentist prepared it, and what it includes. In addition, the receptionists have the option to write a review of the follow up on the plan file itself – "On X, I spoke to Mr. Smith and he asked for a more extensive payment plan; I promised to return to the matter this coming Monday." Every proposal that is closed and in which the client has begun treatment is taken out of the folder. The only files left in the folder are those of clients who have not yet decided on a plan.

It is recommended to take about an hour a day to go over the binder and extract data such as whom you need to call, whether you need to find out more information for the client, etc. Additionally, once a week the receptionists should sit with the dentist or owner and go through the list of proposals that were issued and were not closed, check how each proposal is progressing, and what can be done to close it.

B. **Monitoring chart for treatment plans** – At a certain stage, many treatment plans will accumulate in the binder; this makes it difficult to follow. Therefore, in order to easily find any plan and see all of them at a glance without having to browse through the many programs, a simple table should be prepared, in which you register every checkup. Enter everyone who visited the practice, even if they did not need a treatment plan.

The table will contain only a few important columns: date, client's name, phone number, price of the treatment plan, and comments. With just a glance at the table, you will be able to see the number of exams that require a follow up, so that it will be easy to know what treatment plans to focus on. The comment section should be a sentence or two, summarizing where the monitoring of the treatment plan stands. Most importantly, highlight the treatment plans that have been closed, or those that cannot be closed, so that it will be easy to find treatment programs that require further follow-up.

C. **Timing of the tracking of treatment plans** – The best time to begin follow-ups is two days after a client received the offer. This is a good time both because it was not too long ago that they visited the practice, and because the client has not had time to do much regarding the matter. The continuation of the follow-up will depend on the client's response. For example, the client can say that they have not yet gone to the bank to examine the financial issue, and therefore would like to be in touch in another two weeks. Note this on the proposal and make sure to contact them in about two weeks. However, if client says they have thought about it and decided that they are not interested, you should of course accept this and let them know that if they change their mind they are welcome to contact you at any time.

D. **The script of the follow-up talk should be sensitive and assertive**: "Ms. Green, hello, what can I do in order for you to be treated by us and receive the best treatment?" This seems to be an innocent sentence, but note that it contains several very important and accurate messages. A: "What can I do for you" – means we are not engaged in argument but rather I'm here to help you; and what client will refuse a practice manager or receptionist who wants to help them? B: "You'll get the best treatment" highlights the fact that they will receive the best treatment at your practice.

Four Strategies for Following up on Treatment Plans that Have Not Been Closed

No matter how you look at it, the sale begins the moment the client leaves the practice. After all, most clients take the treatment plan and go home to think about it, consult their acquaintances, etc. From the moment the client leaves the practice to think, every closer of treatment plans must be aware of the options available so that the patients return with a credit card on hand. Of course, each case is different and the strategy chosen depends on the situation and the client. There are four main strategies for bringing back clients who go home to think about a plan.

1. **Solution to medical questions** – In many cases, the client does not really understand the plan: What is a sinus lift? Why didn't the other practice say anything about a bone transplant? And so on and so forth. As long as the client has questions about the medical procedure there is no chance that they will close the deal and start the treatment, and therefore the practice receptionist or manager must answer their questions at least on a basic level. Important tip: in cases such as this, the receptionist or manager of the practice should try to put the client on the phone with the dentist so that the dentist can answer the client's medical questions.

   Even if the receptionist knows what a sinus lift is, it is always better for clients to hear the answers from the dentist. When the client receives a phone call from the dentist who answers their questions, they simultaneously have their questions answered and conclude that this is a service-oriented practice that is very worth joining.

2. **Additional discount or payment plan** – The client wants to be treated by you and they understand the treatment, but just want to pay less. Very nice! Important tip: do not be angry with clients or quarrel with them. They are doing exactly what everyone does, including you. You should hope that you have raised the price enough that you have the option of providing them with what they want. Another important tip: in large treatment plans around $15,000 and upward, it is worthwhile to check the costs of the plan; only then will you really know what the lowest price you can offer is.

   Here, too, acting skills are needed for closing the treatment plan: "Ms. Green, let me see what extra discount I can get for you. I'll talk to the dentist and try to get you a discount from the lab as well."

3. **Offer a more limited program** – The client wants to be treated by you, but it is very expensive for them to undergo an implant treatment for the whole mouth. On the other hand, prosthesis on implants is an option that could suit them and their budget. Important tip: do not ask the client, "What is your budget?" They will never tell you the real budget. Another important tip: never rule out cheap

plans like prosthetics or prosthetics on implants. The strategy should be, "All the treatments are good; you should undergo the treatment you want (as long as you do it here)."

4. **Only deal with urgent matters at this stage** – The client may not have the budget for the program they want, are taking some time to decide, or simply have difficulty deciding. The best strategy in this situation is to create urgency: "You want to think about the plan? OK, no problem! You should, however, take care of the inflammation in the outer area of the lower jaw as soon as possible, and extract the tooth that is pushing on the tooth next to it and could damage it." If you are able to convince the clients to start a small part of the treatment, it is likely that they will continue receiving treatment with you. Important tip: people think in terms of profit and loss; that's why everyone runs to get their car serviced (at the cost of hundreds of dollars) simply because they are afraid of mishaps.

Therefore, the client must understand that if they do not deal with the filling, the situation may deteriorate into a root canal treatment, and if it is not treated, they may even lose the tooth. As soon as they understand this, they will choose preventive treatment.

Key Phrases for Closing Treatment Plans

Each treatment closer must be equipped with key phrases that are important for the closing process. Here are two key and sophisticated phrases that you should retrieve at the right time in order to improve the closing levels of treatment plans.

First sentence: *"Forget the price for a moment; where you would like to undergo the treatment?"*

The client is confused and it is difficult for them to decide. The purpose of this sentence is to separate the economic issue from the medical one and thus simplify the decision. Therefore, the client first has to decide where they want to undergo treatment. You'd be surprised, but that's the essential decision and the most difficult one for them. As soon as the client says – and hears themselves say – "I want to undergo treatment with you," this is a huge advance towards closing the deal, since all that remains is to reach an agreement on the price.

If the client says that they don't know where they want to receive care (there are other dentists who are as good as you are) the focus will be on giving reasons why they should receive care with you – seniority, expertise, stability, etc. – and not conversations about the price.

Second sentence: *"Are we talking about now or later?"* You should use this statement when the client asks for a discount while negotiating a treatment plan. The purpose of this innocent question is to know whether the client is ready to close and start treatment, or whether they are still in the process of receiving quotes from other practices. If the client answers that they want to start care now, then the closer should use the discount to close the deal immediately.

However, if the client responds that they cannot make a decision yet because they have another examination next week, it would be inappropriate to move forward with a final discount. In this case, you should send them on their way with the hope of a maximal discount when they are ripe to make a decision.

Of course, it is necessary to call the client the following week and ask, "What can I do in order for you to receive care with us and get the best treatment," and so on.

How to approach clients who conduct a market survey

You know these clients – those who come to the practice after they have visited several practices, received at least three suggestions for treatment plans, searched Google for all types of implants, prices, and even all the pros and cons of zirconia crowns.

They probably annoy you, do they not?

Well, think again, because if you think of them as pests (as many do) who are only interested in the price, you'll probably treat them as such, and you're sure to lose them!

In fact, if we think logically for a moment, these are your best clients! Why? Because the very fact that they make the rounds in different practices means the most important thing to you: they very much want to undergo the treatment.

One of the biggest and most common mistakes that I see among those who close treatment plans is that they think that these clients go from practice to practice, just looking for the lowest price. This is a false and incorrect assumption – there are clients who buy the first vehicle they like and those who cannot make up their minds until they have tested at least three cars.

Here are six tips that will increase your chances of winning the hearts and pockets of clients who conduct a market survey among several practices.

1. **Encouragement** – First, encourage these clients by letting them know that they are doing the right thing by getting more offers: "Very nice, I'm glad you have other offers. You will be able to really evaluate and understand the treatment plan we are offering you." This way, you can gain their confidence.

2. **Trust** – Clients will choose the practice that wins their trust, expresses the most empathy towards them, and especially, creates a sense of professionalism – where they are offered a detailed proposal, a reasonable plan, and are treated with respect and patience while receiving answers to their questions. Note that these clients are usually confused by the number of proposals they received and therefore the trust you produce is most important.
Another point: do not dismiss the other dentists who offered them other plans

("Who's the cobbler who offered you this plan?") because it might come back to bite you. It can be said implicitly: "Look, there are all kinds of approaches to dentistry. I don't know whom you got suggestions from and it doesn't really matter, but with us, there are no shortcuts." (Which clients will want shortcuts when it comes to dental treatments?) "It is no accident that we have been preforming dental implants for 15 years, and that our success rate stands at about 96% [if this is true]."

3. **"So what if you have cheaper offers?"** – Do not worry about clients receiving cheaper offers. Instead, you need to ask yourself why the clients came to you if they have a cheaper offer. Why didn't they go to the cheap practice? Well, the answer is simple: they are probably afraid of the cheap offer they received, since clients think that cheap means low quality and expensive means high quality. In fact, clients who come back to you after receiving a cheaper offer from a different practice just want another small discount in order to close the deal with you. You should hope that you adjusted for the final discount of closing the transaction.

As I have mentioned, clients are not looking for the cheapest price; they are afraid of prices that are too cheap, but are looking for the cheapest price they can get from you! This, or at least the feeling that they will get the lowest price possible, is what you must provide.

4. **Avoid point-to-point comparisons** – Beware of point-to-point comparisons with other, cheap offers. If you compare information in this way, you will communicate that you are the same. Just say, "Mr. Smith, in dentistry, as in any other field, there are all kinds of price levels. At our practice's level of professionalism, and considering our standards–" (here I recommend adding the competitive advantages of the practice: medical expertise, years of experience, training, innovative and advanced equipment, etc.) "–these are the prices. There are less expensive and more expensive prices, and you are entitled to choose what standard of care you want to receive."

In certain situations, it is advisable to add the following sentence: "It is not that we earn more; we simply have a high level of treatment and materials that come at higher costs. There is no such thing as high quality at a low cost. What you should compare point-to-point is the medical treatment program. Mr. Smith, I find it difficult to understand how you were offered treatment without a bone graft, when you have no bone at all. What will the implants be attached to?"

5. **Maximum coverage** – Offer these clients two or three alternatives to a treatment plan. Why? Because if you only offer an implant plan for $60,000 they may not be able to afford it, and if they receive an offer from another dentist for a prosthesis on implants at $35,000, it is reasonable to assume that they will turn to the other dentist for treatment rather than to you. The goal is for the client to undergo whatever program they want and can finance – with you. In addition, it is easier for clients to make a decision on what is good for them when they have two or three alternatives, instead of only one option.

6. **Goodbye, but not farewell** – If the client has not completed the rounds at other practices, you should come to two conclusions with them before you part ways, provided you have developed trust and friendship. A: "Before you make a final decision, come to us for another consultation so we can give you an opinion on the treatment plan you want to perform and make sure it is medically correct." B: "Once you have definitively decided that you want to carry out the treatment plan, I will work for you to get another discount."

PART FOUR

ATTRACTING NEW CLIENTS TO THE PRACTICE

Chapter 13

How to Attract New Clients to the Practice

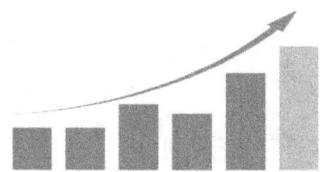

In my lectures, I present a slide with the question, *What are the three factors that most influence the success of a dental practice?* The participants usually give brief and predictable answers such as: the quality of the treatments, quality of the staff, and location of the practice. Then I present the next slide with the answer:

1. New exams
2. New exams
3. New exams

This is not a joke; it's reality. It's all about statistics: more exams mean more treatment plans closed. A dental practice with the best dentists, best location, etc., but with only a few new exams per month, will not be successful. On the other hand, a practice that is mid-level in terms of the dentists' quality and the treatments but manages to set up appointments for many exams is more likely to be more successful. Ideally, of course, your practice will uphold the highest standards in all parameters, as well as procure many new tests.

It really doesn't matter whether the new exams are for long-standing clients or new ones; what matters is that the examination takes place and leads to a treatment plan. There are two main sources for increasing the number of new exams at the practice. The first is through existing customers, which I discussed at length in the chapter on customer retention and cultivation of recommenders. This chapter will focus on the second source of increasing the number of exams in the practice: gaining new customers, with a key element in getting new clients to the practice being advertising.

Advertising the Practice

One of the most troublesome issues any dental practice owner has is advertising. Since this is a broad and complex subject, I will focus on the six most fundamental questions related to advertising: Is it worthwhile to advertise the dental practice? Does advertising lead to a lesser image of the practice? How should we invest in advertising? What should we advertise? Where should we advertise? How can you test the effectiveness of advertising?

Should you advertise?

I'll get straight to the bottom line: not only is it worthwhile to advertise, but you must advertise! Why? Simple because, at this very moment, there are hundreds of people who need dental treatment, living near your practice. Some may need small treatments but some need larger treatments, like complete oral rehab. Wouldn't you want them to come in for treatment at your practice? Wouldn't you at least want them to come in for a consultation and exam with you? That's why you set up your practice, wasn't it?

Guess what? There is only one small thing that separates you from the people who live in the vicinity and need dental care; they simply do not know that your practice exists. If they do not know that your practice exists, then the fact that your practice is amazing and uses the most innovative methods is irrelevant because unfortunately treatments are being performed elsewhere.

Therefore, the primary function of advertising is to inform your potential target audience that you exist. By the way, to remove any doubt – there is no other way to inform your audience that you exist except to use mass media channels. Believe me, companies do not enjoy spending a lot of money on advertising, but they do; they have no other choice and in the end, it pays off financially.

Does Advertising Damage the Practice's Image?

Definitely not! As long as you advertise in a respectable and ethical manner and according to the rules of the Ministry of Health (without displaying prices, promotions, false information, etc.) or according to local regulations, advertising does not damage your image. Today there is no commercial field that does not advertise. The competition is huge in all sectors of the market – and certainly in dental care – so there are not many choices but to advertise. As stated, the goal is simply to inform the audience of your practice's existence.

The idea that advertising creates a cheap image is a relic of veteran dentists for whom, 25 years ago and more, the intensity of competition was minor, and advertising medical services was indeed unacceptable. However, as we know, the rules of the game have changed and anyone who wants to survive the competition should play the game as it is currently played.

How much should you invest in advertising?

There is no exact answer to this question, but companies tend to allocate a certain percentage of their revenue to advertising. The percentage varies according to the field, market, and other business variables. In my experience, the optimal percentage for the dental care field is 3-5% of sales. This percentage should be weighed with additional variables, for example, a new practice will spend a higher percentage on advertising than an established one; a practice that focuses on full oral rehabilitation treatments, where profits are higher, will also spend a higher percentage of the profit on advertising.

It is important to remember that advertising is like coals: you need to fan them constantly so that they don't go out. A practice that is supported by regular advertising will gain a greater influx of new patients and a higher sales cycle. It's true that investing in advertising does increase spending, but if advertising is performed correctly, it generally also increases revenue and profitability. Incidentally, advertising also works for customer retention – it reminds existing customers that you exist.

What about the return on investment? A well-known saying goes: "The only thing that is known about advertising is how much you spend." You'll never know what your return on investment will be for advertising; but in my experience, if you advertise using the right channels with the right message and allocate the right percentage, in the vast majority of cases, not only will you make a return on the investment but you will also make a big profit.

In practice, most dental practices do not have a defined advertising budget, which is a pity. Have no doubt – a practice does not save money by not advertising. On the contrary, it loses money by not investing in advertising or informing potential customers of its existence, and as a result, they do not come and close treatment plans.

I tend to offer dental practices that have difficulty spending money on advertising the following advice: raise prices by 5% and allocate the same 5% of the turnover to advertising. Customers will continue to come to you for care even after the price increases, and you will have an advertising budget with which to increase the circle of new customers.

What should you advertise?

The main message of the campaign should be derived from the goals set by the practice. In any case, before you start building your message, you should read up on any advertising restrictions and ethics that apply to dentists, and act accordingly. However, it is worth noting several points in building the message:

A. **Beware of multiple messages** – A well-known rule in marketing and advertising is, "Here and there is neither here nor there." If you try to convey many messages, you will not communicate anything. If the defined campaign goals are to increase the number of transplants, it is best to focus on transplants rather than to advertise the fact that a new orthodontist has joined the practice.

B. **The dentist is the brand** – It is easier for potential customers to reach out to the practice once they know whom the dentists are and what they look like. Clients can connect to a dentist's picture more easily than to a dentist's name. In addition, an image of the dentists in the ad should remind customers of their existence. A veteran practice team – receptionists, assistants, hygienists – should also add their pictures, to add humanity and warmth to the practice's image.

C. **Professionalism** – It is worthwhile to emphasize all the competitive advantages of the practice, such as seniority, expertise, and training in prestigious schools. Don't forget that this is the most important factor for customers when they choose a practice.

D. **Aesthetic design** – Advertising medical services must be done in a clean and aesthetic way. Your advertising is your image – if you post beautiful and aesthetic ads, this will broadcast that the practice performs aesthetic and beautiful treatments. This, of course, works in the opposite direction as well. In addition, it is worthwhile to remember that the ads are supposed to convey calm and confidence (certain colors can achieve this, for example green, light blue, and blue). In any case, it is worthwhile to hire a graphic designer who specializes in the nuances of advertising medical services.

Where Should You Advertise?

There are several possible channels for a practice to reach new customers. The choice as to which channel(s) should be used depends on many factors, since a channel that fits practice X is not necessarily right for practice Y. I have come across cases where a particular channel worked very well for one practice, but did not work at all for another practice. What should be done, then? The answer is – try! If you have advertised using a certain channel a number times and have not received enough inquiries, move on to the next channel until you reach the most effective channel for you: the one that produces quality inquiries.

Here are the possible channels of action for acquiring new customers.

A. Local press

Until recently, the local press was considered the most popular advertising channel for dental practices for two main reasons: advertising costs are relatively low, and in most cases, the geographical area closest to the practice is the primary target audience. However, it is important to remember that the printed press is now in constant decline – readership has moved to digital media. However, there are areas (especially in suburbs) where local, veteran newspapers will not die out so quickly, especially among the aging audience, therefore this is definitely a worthy channel for a practice to try.

It is worth noting that although ads in the local press will not produce a flood of phone calls, it is worth examining their effectiveness according to the number of treatments they have generated for the practice following the publication and not the number of calls.

Here's a real case: One of the practices I visited launched a one-month campaign in the local press, with an investment of several hundred dollars. To our disappointment, the campaign yielded only 15 phone calls. To our delight, one of the new customers closed a treatment plan worth $30,000! (Two jaw treatments including everything!) Another closed a $3,000 treatment plan – a worthwhile investment by all accounts. When choosing to advertise in the local press, advertising should not be a one-off deal, rather, it is recommended to spread it out over time. You will not always get reactions to the first publication; sometimes it takes time for the target audience to digest the ad.

Additionally, it's best for the same ad to appear throughout the advertising period rather than be replaced every week – consistency is important when it comes to advertising, since the customers are not the enemy and therefore there is no need to confuse them.

B. Public Relations

There is no doubt that PR is one of the most effective channels for the dentists and the practice, and no less importantly – it is free. All that is required is to initiate press releases in local newspapers or social media about the dentist and/or practice. Did the dentist attend a dental conference? Did you care for a famous client? Did you celebrate a receptionist's birthday? Take a picture, write a few words, and send it (with the click of a mouse) to the newspaper or post it on the practice's social media accounts. It is also possible to initiate something more professional such as a regular column on the subject of dentistry, written in an accessible style: What is orthodontic treatment? Is toothpaste harmful to teeth? Tips for effective brushing. And so on.

In this way, potential customers in the area will read about you once, twice, and a third time, and in the end will make the connection and come to the conclusion, "This this is a good dentist!". At a certain practice, we ran a PR campaign that focused on the practice's medical director. After a few months, in which we focused on the dentist's professionalism and gradually sent out local press reports, the number of new customers for implants treatments increased significantly.

Another point that should be made clear is that when you advertise regularly in a local newspaper, they develop a kind of commitment to you. Therefore, when you want to publish an article about your participation at a surgical conference abroad, or if you win a professional award, it is reasonable to assume that the same newspaper will not refuse to publish about you because they do not want to lose you as an advertiser.

C. Direct mail

Customers usually prefer that their dentist be close to their home or place of work, for two reasons. First, convenience: it is easier for the clients to receive treatment in a practice close to their home or workplace. Second, in case the customers need an emergency appointment, it will be simple and quick for them to get to the practice.

This is why it is highly recommended that all residents in the general vicinity of the practice know that you exist.

One of the most effective ways to inform residents and professionals in the area of the practice's presence is through direct mail. This is a relatively small expense, including only an envelope, stationery, and a selection of the practice's brochures.

It is worthwhile to address the residents or professionals in a personal, short, and matter-of-fact manner, and emphasize the fact that the practice is close to their home or workplace, in the following style: "Dear resident of Main Street; many people prefer that their dentist be close to their home or workplace. It is more convenient and sometimes, unfortunately, we need an emergency appointment. I wanted to inform you that there is a dental practice specializing in ___ on Christopher Street, close to your home."

In addition to emphasizing the proximity of the dental practice, direct mailing must offer bait that will motivate clients to approach the practice at least once, such as, "Dr. Kumar's Practice offers unique benefits for residents/professionals in the area during the next two months, including free exams and plaque removal. You are invited to contact us today to schedule an appointment."

As stated, the request should be personal, brief, and matter-of-fact. Residents can read about the practice and the types of treatments provided in the attached brochure. Direct mail distribution should be carried out by the post office or direct mail companies that specialize in distributing advertising materials.

Response to direct mail is very low, but it's all about statistics – if you fill mailboxes with thousands of fliers (inside a closed envelope), it is very likely that you will reach residents who happen to be looking for a dentist. It is important to note that the use of the direct mailing channel is not the preferred option in most cases, but in some cases, we were very surprised by the results, especially in small residential areas that make more use of mailboxes.

D. Reaching out to workplaces in an organized manner

Many practices are located in areas where there are many businesses (offices, large stores, etc.), mainly in city centers. As mentioned in the previous section, people prefer their dentist to be close to their workplace, since there is nothing more convenient then having plaque removed or a filling done during your lunch hour or right after work. Reaching out to workplaces around the practice may add a large number of new customers – not only local professionals but their families as well.

However, turning to workplaces in the area requires proper preparation. Adding professionals to your client list requires building a good and attractive infrastructure and investing many hours of work; however, this is a worthwhile investment. Recruiting customers from a number of offices and factories in the area may increase the number of customers significantly. For example, a single accounting firm with 12 employees may add up to 30 potential clients to the practice, if you consider their families. Now calculate how many offices there are in the area and how you can increase the number of customers at your practice.

It is important to emphasize another matter in this context: both your practice and the workplaces in the area will profit. On the one hand, people love to take advantage of size and make centralized purchases to achieve good purchasing value. On the other hand, the practice is interested in a large number of customers and in return, it is ready give up a certain percentage of profit. This is the guiding principle of all connections between places of work and commercial bodies.

How do you do this? In several stages

Step 1 – Establish a unique membership club for the practice, which workplaces can join. The club will include special benefits for members such as free membership, free examinations, a certain discount on all treatments, free emergency appointments, and one dental cleaning a year at a special price.

Step 2 – Segment businesses located in the area and make a list of those that should be contacted. For example, the practice may decide that it only appeals to law firms, accounting firms, and high-tech companies. By the way, the breakdown of businesses close to the practice can be obtained from companies that deal with such databases, or by legwork.

Step 3 – The practice representative contacts the selected workplaces and requests to meet with the CEO or business owner: "I'd be happy to meet with you for 20 minutes in order to offer you unique benefits that we have developed for the area's professionals." The practice will be presented at the meeting (preferably through the brochure or its website and maybe even through a visit to the practice) and the representative will discuss the unique benefits that the practice offers to professionals in the area. It is worth noting that the CEO or company have nothing to lose, since they will be perceived as caring for their employees.

Step 4 – If the CEO or business owner expresses interest in the membership club, all that is required is to issue a personal letter on their behalf and with their signature (although the practice should prepare the text), to the employees. The text should be as follows: "Dear employee; I'm happy to inform you that we have reached an arrangement with the X dental practice, located close to the office, on Y Street. Membership is free and offers unique benefits such as X% discount on all treatments, an exam plus two X-rays for free," and so on.

It should also be noted in the letter that membership is not binding and is a recommendation only, in order to remove any responsibility from the CEO or business owner and prevent them from worrying about making a recommendation to their employees.

It should also be noted in the letter that, "When setting up the appointment employees must mention that they are members of the club and bring their membership card to their appointment." The letter will also note that, "Families of employees will be entitled to the same benefits upon presentation of the card." Leverage the club membership in order to recruit as many new customers as possible.

Step 5 – The letter from the CEO or business owner, the practice's brochure, and membership card will be placed in an envelope and distributed to employees.

Step 6 – Separate registration and follow-up with club members: how many treatments did they undergo, how much revenue did the practice produce from the club members, and how much was invested in them? I would like to emphasize that it is reasonable to assume that some members of the club will only take advantage of the benefits and seemingly be a burden on the practice. However, statistically, some of them will also carry out treatments that may not only return the investment, but also generate profits for the practice.

An important insight: the model presented above works very well. Practices I have accompanied in this type of process managed to recruit hundreds of new customers exactly according to this method. Not all employees join – some have a dentist who they are not willing to part with, but a considerable number of employees are happy to receive such a benefit. There is only one danger to this method: if a club member from a particular workplace does not receive good service, the information spreads like wildfire among all the club members at that workplace. The good news is that it works the other way around too.

A further insight: the same model can be applied to the committees of large buildings, where the building manager is the "CEO". There are often large buildings near practices that can be explored for cooperation with tenants who will join the practice's members club.

E. Digital Marketing

Don't be confused: digital marketing is mentioned at the end of the chapter on how to recruit new clients, but in the work plan of any dental practice it should be a top priority. Why? In recent years, and probably in the coming years, this is the most effective channel for recruiting new customers.

What is digital marketing? There are many interpretations to this question, but in general, this is a comprehensive definition of all Internet channels – websites, search engines (like Google), and social networks (like Facebook, Instagram, and Twitter), and so on.

Digital marketing is developing at a very fast pace thanks to smart phones, which enable customers to search and gather information with amazing ease, anywhere and at any given moment. The result? More and more customers do not spend money before they search the Internet. If clients understand that they should perform dental implants, they will immediately search Google for information about dental implants: who performs the procedure, how it is done, and how much it costs. Even if someone's friend recommended you, he or she will type your name into Google and search for information about you. The worst thing that can happen is for customers to find nothing about you and your practice.

I will not go into detail here about the tactical level of how to perform digital marketing, for the simple reason that the digital world is so dynamic that it's likely that everything I write on the matter may be irrelevant in a short while. Therefore, I'll focus on a basic marketing strategy for digital marketing that should guide you and through which you can build a digital marketing system at any given time.

Here are some guidelines for effective use of digital marketing:

1. **Online Presence** – It is reasonable to assume that customers who live in a certain city and understand the need to care for their teeth will turn to a popular search engine (like Google) and search for "dentist in New York," "dental practice in New York," or something along these lines. The most important question you should ask yourself is whether you appear in the search results. Is the first result (or among the first) the name of your practice and website – or your competitor's?

So, first, let's conduct a short exercise. Step into the shoes of clients who live in the area of your practice and are searching the web for a dentist who performs the treatments you perform, and see if they find you.

Let's say your practice is located in New York and most of your activity is in dental implants and oral rehabilitation. Search the web for "Transplants in New York." What comes up in the results? If you do not appear among the first results this is a problem, because there is no chance that these customers will visit your practice, and that is really too bad.

It's important to point out a basic issue of digital marketing: nothing is coincidental; only those who work on digital marketing will appear first in the search results, as this is the main way for huge companies to make money, and a lot of it.

Another online search should interest you. John, your client, has advised his friend to receive care with you. Guess what his friend immediately does? You guessed it: he goes online and searches for your name. What search results come up when customers do this? After all, from this moment they begin to build the puzzle at the end of which they will decide whether they should turn to you for care. Will the search results lead to an impressive and innovative site with detailed information about the pra c tice's competitive advantages, and an interview with you in a newspaper plus a video of a TV talk show in which you participated, which will get the prospective clients thinking, "Wow, this seems like an impressive dentist"?

Or, as so often happens, the customers' search will not lead to any information on you, which will make them think, "Wait a minute, if John claims that this dentist is so good, how is it that there is no mention of him/her on the Internet?" Sometimes an e ven worse scenario occurs: the first search result is a lawsuit against the dentist; it really does not matter whether the lawsuit is justified or not, and what happened at the end of the trial. This is definitely an unpromising start and creates a problematic first impression of the dentist, who may have been wrongly sued.

2. **Digital Marketing Content** – Following the previous section, you should and can control the content that appears online. You will not have a website if you do not bother to build it and there will be no interview if you do not make it happen. On the other hand, a dentist is not a PR person who sits and feeds information to the media all day.

Therefore, do not overdo it with content, but you should make sure that there is at least some essential information about you and the practice, for example, a detailed website including your resume (education, training, years of experience, types of treatments performed, and so on) and that of the additional dentists who work at the practice. You do not have to add too much. Many make the mistake of flooding a website with a great deal of tedious information about the types of implants and treatments, thus confusing the clients. The site should not try to teach the clients dentistry, but rather be simple, user-friendly, and convey that this is a professional, innovative, and reliable practice. In most cases, only a few seconds are enough for whoever is browsing the site to decide whether this practice is one that should be consulted and visited, and therefore all the most important information (seniority, expertise, etc.) should be presented in the first few seconds of browsing the site.

By the way, there is a big advantage in the digital world that should be exploited. Any positive publicity about you or your practice that goes online (interview, article, video, etc.) will be available to prospective customers for years to come. This is in contrast to advertising in the printed press, which expires as soon as the newspaper is thrown away. Therefore, this is an investment for both the present and the distant future.

3. **Measuring the effectivity of the digital campaign** – Another advantage of digital marketing is the ability to measure results more accurately. If you post an ad in the newspaper, you can only guess how many people have been exposed to it. On the other hand, when you advertise on social media, you get accurate data: how many people viewed the ad, how many clicked, how many times it was shared, etc. If you use a mailing list, you can get a report about who opened the email, who clicked the link, what time this happened, how long visits to the site lasted, and how many times a link was clicked.

These help the advertiser get a clearer picture of the effectivity of advertising and make necessary changes accordingly. This is in contrast to traditional advertising, where decisions are made mainly based on intuition rather than precise data.

Still, the most important factor is how much money was invested in the campaign and how much money it made in return. See further details below.

4. **Addressing digital marketing leads** – At the end of the day, many digital marketing campaigns focus on generating leads: contacting customers via email or a landing page. I have encountered practices that used these leads to set up examinations, which eventually increased the practice's sales turnover. However, I have also come across practices that did not handle incoming leads properly, and turned the campaign into a waste of money.

   Here are some important tactical tips for handling leads effectively:

   A. **Documenting leads** – For leads that arrived through the site, do not call them until they are listed in a simple, dedicated Excel sheet that includes the following columns: date, name, phone number, and comments. Tracking will be much more effective through the table than email. In the table, you can briefly list how the follow-up is going for each lead: "Asked us to talk tomorrow," or, "Looking for a gum specialist," and so on.

   B. **When to address the lead** – Did the lead arrive today? It is advisable to contact the customer immediately or the next day at the latest. Two days is a long time; if you contact them more than a day after receiving the lead, there is a possibility that they will no longer remember the matter. Therefore, you should get in touch with customers as quickly as possible when their message to you is still fresh in their mind.

   C. **How to handle a lead** – In quite a few cases, customers who turn to the practice have important questions: Does the practice use general anesthesia? Are there specialists at the practice? How many sessions are needed for straightening teeth? And so on. The manner in which the receptionists answer customers' questions will determine whether customers will want to come to the practice. Impatient responses will cause customers to move on to the next practice, but a patient and empathic response will communicate that this is a professional practice that will make them feel safe to come in for a checkup. Therefore, it is imperative to take time and address leads, and concentrate solely on the phone conversation with the prospective clients, since the sales process begins at this stage. Addressing leads from the receptionists' desk in the middle of ongoing work is an anticipated failure.

D. **Creating a sense of urgency regarding exams** – One of the biggest drawbacks of digital marketing is that in some cases inquiries are received from customers with a low level of urgency, who do not show up to the appointment they set up. ("I waited this long to go to a dentist; nothing will happen if I do not show up.") One of the most effective solutions for increasing the percentage of arrivals is to create a sense of urgency with potential clients.

How do you do this? During the phone conversation, the client describes the reason for their contact: "One of my back teeth fell out about two years ago and I want to see what you can do about it." Just setting up an appointment, without creating urgency, could create a situation in which the appointment will be postponed if the smallest thing comes up; after all, he has been walking around without a back tooth for two years.

However, if the receptionist produces a (quite realistic) sense of urgency in the following style: "Mr. Smith, it is not recommended to walk around with a missing tooth. In cases such as these, there is a movement of the teeth in the mouth to fill the void created by the missing tooth. Many teeth can be hurt in this process, which is a shame. I advise you not to neglect this and come to see what Dr. Jones can do about it," there is no doubt that Mr. Smith will think twice before deciding to cancel his appointment.

5. **Find a good digital marketer** – As mentioned above, digital marketing evolves very quickly, and constant updating is required in order to perform it best. A dentist is supposed to practice medicine and not digital marketing, and therefore, you should hire the services of a digital marketing expert who will do the work for you. The digital marketing expert knows all the methods and is up-to-date on the news, and therefore can do a good and effective job for you, so that you can focus on what you are best at: dentistry.

However, even if you hire a digital marketing specialist, it is strongly recommended that you participate in a crash course or lecture, or even read a related book, in order to have a general understanding of digital marketing. You cannot afford not to know anything about the most important marketing tool that should be advancing your career and financial situation.

It's worth noting that not everything is rosy in the field. Unfortunately, because anyone with a computer and an Internet connection can present themselves as a digital marketing expert, there are quite a few amateurs and even charlatans in the field – both individuals and companies.

While choosing a digital marketing person or company, you should pay attention to a number of important things, in order for the investment to pay off and not become an unnecessary waste of money.

A. Do not to commit to a contract for a certain period. If there are no results during the first three months, there will be none in the next few months; so why pay for a whole year? You should monitor how much you pay and what you get in return, and if there are no positive results terminate the engagement immediately.

B. You must demand complete transparency from the marketing people as to how much of the budget goes to them in order to manage the campaign, and how much of the budget goes to pay media channels. Theoretically, a marketing person can allocate most of the budget to himself while the not leaving enough money to pay media channels to reach your target audience.

C. It is necessary to receive a monthly report from the digital marketing experts: what was the expense and which results were gained in terms of exposure, number of leads, and so on.

D. Dental marketing has its own rules and nuances. Therefore, you should hire the services of those who understand the field of dental marketing. A general marketing person who does not know the difference between a specialist and a general dentist, or what it means to complete dental implants in one day, will probably not be able to build an effective campaign for you.

Measuring advertising effectivity

It is not easy to measure the effect of advertising and its direct impact on sales. I believe that the only thing that can be accurately measured in advertising is how much money is paid for it. The difficulty in measuring the effect of advertising stems from the fact that the advertisement has direct effects that can be easily measured, for example, a customer who calls and says "Hello, I saw your post and I want to set up an appointment," etc. However, many indirect effects cannot be measured precisely.

For example, dormant clients who have not visited the practice for eight years and are suddenly exposed to the practice's publicity and call to schedule an appointment will be cataloged as existing customers rather than new ones attracted by publicity initiatives, even though it is highly doubtful that they would have called had they not been exposed to this. Or, dormant clients awakened by advertising who later advise their friends about the practice; the friend will be categorized as someone who came by word of mouth and not through advertising, and so on.

Despite the complexity, each practice must try to measure the effectiveness of advertising to make correct strategic decisions. There are two ways to measure the effectiveness of advertising. The first is to ask new customers how they arrived at the practice and keep an accurate record, so that through a quick assessment you can tell how many of them came due to advertising, and how much money came in as a result. Following this, compare the revenues from customers who arrived through advertising to the financial investment that the practice spent on advertising, and receive a picture of the advertising investment's profitability. Of course, the indirect effects of advertising, which cannot be measured and weighed, should be taken into account.

The second way to help you complete the picture about advertising effectiveness is to compare sales turnover during the period of advertising with the previous sales turnover. Good publicity should affect the sales graph; if the graph does not move, then the advertising is probably not effective. On the other hand, if there is a sudden significant jump in sales in the same period in which you began advertising, even if no customers say that they came following the advertising, it is worth continuing to advertise and even increase your ad budget.

These two tests can give you a general idea of the effectiveness of advertising. Though it is not accurate, a general picture can help you make the right decision about advertising: Should you continue advertising? Increase or decrease your budget? And so on. Based on the vast experience I have accumulated in advertising dental practices as part of the business consulting I provide, I can say that advertising most definitely works, and in any case, there is no other option but to advertise. You have a dental practice and in order for patients to visit it, they need to know that it exists. And there is no way besides advertising that you can use to inform the public of the practice's existence.

PART FIVE

THE PRACTICE'S BUSINESS CONDUCT

Chapter 14

Realizing the Practice's Potential

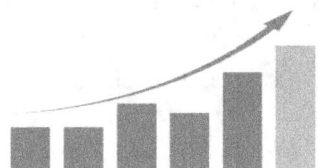

Although every practice is interested in realizing its potential for sales turnover and profitability, in practice, only a few dental practices succeed when it comes to this task. Why? Because in order to be as successful as possible, the practice should function perfectly both strategically and tactically – and this is not a simple thing to do.

Since it is difficult to achieve perfect function that will bring about the realization of maximum potential, the question is, how much of its potential does your practice manage to realize? Is it 80% or only about 40%? Well, let me tell you a little secret: The vast majority of practices realize 40% of their potential or even less. It is no accident that in my marketing consulting process, I manage to double the sales cycles of many practices within a relatively short time.

Before I deal with the issues that prevent dental practices from realizing their potential, it is worth noting the main factors affecting sales potential and a practice's profitability.

1. **Combination of treatments** – The more the practice provides surgical and reconstructive services (transplants, sinus lifts, etc.) and fewer preservative treatments (fillings, root canal treatments, etc.), the higher the sales turnover and profitability per unit will be, and vice versa. I know of many dental practices with full appointment books and high productivity, but whose sales turnover and profitability are low because most of the treatments performed there are unprofitable.

2. **Seniority** – Of course, a one- or two-year-old practice will not succeed in realizing a higher percentage of its potential. However, a practice with about seven years' seniority in the same location should be realizing or at least approaching its potential.

3. **Location** – The practice's location has a major impact on the sales cycle and especially the size of the target audience in the area. Practices located in big cities with a larger consumer base will find it easier to achieve their business potential than practices located in remote areas, even though practices located in the suburbs have other advantages such as lower costs, less competition, and so on.

Chapter 15

Recommended Business Strategy

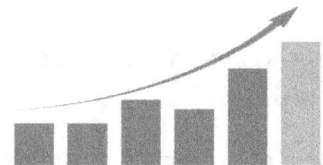

The marketing strategy of a practice that succeeds in getting close to realizing its potential should be, "Preserving what exists," which includes mainly marketing and customer retention activities to maintain the current level of income. Maintaining the status quo sounds simple in theory, but in reality, success is fluid and changing, and there is truth in the saying, "It's easier to achieve success than to keep it."

A practice that is far from realizing its potential should examine itself and perform improvements in several areas. Below are some issues that may prevent a practice from exercising its potential.

1. **An unsuitable team** – Receptionists who do not know how to provide service and cause many matters to fall between the cracks, treatment plan closers that do not know how to sell, slow or indifferent dentists, and so on.

2. **Incorrect pricing** – The practice charges prices that are either lower or higher than it should.

3. **Professionalism** – Low-level dentistry that creates negative word of mouth and discourages recommendations and new customers.

4. **New appointments** – Lack of new patients at the practice. A practice cannot reach high sales cycles without new exams.

5. **Sales** – Low treatment plan closing percentages due to an incorrect or unprofessional sales chain.

6. **Customer retention** – Poor customer retention such as failure to maintain contact with customers or defective implementation of the RE-CALL system.

7. **Customer service** – Incorrect marketing and administrative policies such as the management of appointments, collection, and discounts.

8. **Organizational structure** – Failure in the practice's organizational structure, problematic division of responsibilities, poor management, lack of work force, and so on.

9. **Motivation** – The practice's employees are embittered and not motivated to succeed and promote the practice.

10. **Initial testing** – Customers are given suggestions for incorrect treatment plans (from a marketing perspective).

11. **Follow up** – There is no systematic follow-up of treatment plans that have not been closed.

12. **Internal marketing** – Lack of marketing activities aimed at the practice's customer base.

13. **Poor branding** – Lack of marketing and branding activities, which result in a low positioning of the practice, for example, an old-fashioned and unprofessional appearance.

In conclusion, there is a direct connection between the practice's level of functioning and the realization of sales potential and profitability. Its sales cycles and level of profitability attest to a practice's function more than anything else does.

In my marketing and consulting work, the sales cycle is the main parameter for building a work plan for a practice. The equation is very simple: high sales cycles and high profitability attest to the good functioning of the practice and therefore an "improvement strategy" is required – an improvement in the number of new exams, improving the professional perception of the practice, and so on.

On the other hand, when I encounter low sales and profitability cycles, it is clear to me that this is a case of a malfunction in essential matters at the practice, and therefore, a more aggressive and revolutionary strategy is required in order to bring about a change in the sales turnover. This is, of course, only after I have identified which deficiencies are causing the low sales cycles.

It may sound obvious, but in my consulting work, I have encountered quite a few practice owners that do not understand this simple equation. For example, a practice owner whose sales turnover is high but is not satisfied with the team's performance and believes that they are not good enough at their jobs. How is it possible that the team is not good enough if sales cycles are high? After all, the team plays a considerable part in a practice's ability to reach high sales cycles. Alternatively, a practice whose sales turnover is low but the owner is absolutely sure that everything is done correctly.

The problem is that when you do not follow this equation you usually find yourself making wrong decisions and causing damage to the practice. I've seen too many practice owners who are sure they are doing everything just right and that their sales turnover is low because of competition with public practices, or because of the recession, etc. If only they understood that the sales cycle is a mirror of the practice's function, they might look inward, identify the failures, correct them, and improve the sales cycles.

Chapter 16

The Practice's Financial Conduct

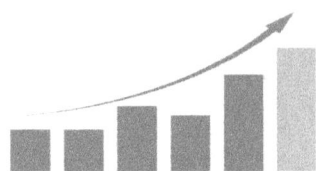

Proper financial conduct is one of the most important things for a practice's success. However, unfortunately I have come across quite a few practices that are able to generate high sales volumes but are in cash flow distress due to erroneous financial conduct.

Cash flow distress in the practice's bank account directly affects the practice's function. The owner becomes stressed and frustrated, the practice cannot invest in advertising and marketing, there is nothing to talk about in terms of raising employees' wages, no money for new equipment, and so on and so forth. All this leads to a negative loop, which makes the practice a helpless hostage to its problematic bank account.

A dental practice should not be cash flow distress if it is managed properly and does not go on unnecessary adventures – and certainly when the practice manages to generate reasonable revenues.

Here are some important points of financial management that will help you keep your bank account steady and out of debt.

1. **There is no connection between practice profitability and cash flow distress** – The practice can be very profitable and have a large overdraft at the same time. To use a simple equation, you can make a million dollars a month but if you spend a million and a half, you will be half a million overdrawn. Yes, simple math – it not only matters how much you put in, it's also important how much you spend. The practice owner's attitude is very important here; there are people

who will buy a device for $5,000 only when they have $15,000, and there are those who would like to buy the device for $5,000 when they have only $1,000 available. Guess who has a much greater chance of being in cash flow distress? You guessed it.

2. **Absolute separation between bank accounts** – One of the most common mistakes of practices that reach cash flow distress is the fact that the business bank account is shared with a private account. In such a situation, you will never know what the business's real financial situation is. Make it a rule to manage the business account and the private account separately – all expenses and revenues from the practice should be managed in the business account. There should be no mixing between the accounts: separate credit cards, separate checks, and completely separate accounts.

The only connection between the accounts is that once a month, on a fixed date, a fixed salary will be transferred (possibly even by standing order) from the business account to the private account. At the end of the year, or even once every six months, you can see whether the business account has "gained weight" and withdraw funds for private needs, but then you can at least see a clear picture of the practice's financial situation. By the way, do not involve business with business! If you own other businesses or another practice, every business should have its own separate account.

3. **The credit trap** – In theory it sounds great: instead of paying $100,000 now, the amount is divided into ten payments and money remains available to the practice. There is only one small problem – you look at the account and you think you have money and allow yourself to buy more equipment, make renovations, etc., but actually the money does not exist – it's fictional because there are many burdensome payments in the background to which you have already committed. Then comes a holiday or, heaven forbid, a recession; the account begins to go red and the phone call from the bank will soon follow.

Do not fool yourself – make it a habit to pay as much cash as possible, and much less in credit and installments. This way you will know exactly where you stand and what your real financial situation is. What's the point of paying the lab in installments? Will there be no lab expenses next month? When you pay in cash, you get an accurate picture of your finances and are able to act accordingly.

When you use credit, you do not know your exact situation and in most cases, you think it is better than it really is. A bit of pessimism is not bad for proper financial conduct.

4. **Controlling expenses** – Following the previous section, buy only with what you have and not with what you don't. It is true that it is more convenient when there is a panoramic camera in the practice, and that if you buy the space next door the practice will be more spacious. Nevertheless, only do it if you actually have the money for it. You can do without a panoramic device in the practice, but it is impossible to manage when there is cash flow distress in the bank account. There are many gadgets in the dental market that cost too much; there is no end to this. First invest in what brings in the patients, and only after there are enough patients, let yourself buy the gadgets. I know a lot of practices that have too many gadgets (which are barely used) and too few customers. An important insight: do not economize on what increases the practice's income directly, for example advertising, or bonuses for treatment plan closers.

5. **Expense Monitoring** – Materials and lab expenses are approximately 20% of turnover, and this is no small expense. Saving a percent or two on this expenditure can amount to a significant sum at the end of the year. What happens in most dental practices is that orders are carried out on a regular and automatic basis, without checking prices. It is very worthwhile to occasionally examine prices and receive quotes from various suppliers you've worked with before; sometimes you can buy the same materials for less money. In addition, it is not advisable to be tempted into inventory sales. Suppliers have very good reasons for wanting you to have a large inventory of their products, but your interest is to have liquid money instead of stock on the practice's shelves.

6. **Additional Matters** –
   A. Make sure that you do not have collection problems at the practice as this may significantly change your entire financial situation.
   B. Make sure you have fair agreements with the dentists you employ since this means you are making some money on the treatments they perform (after lab expenses, materials, assistants, etc.).
   C. Make sure you achieve profitability, not only high productivity.

Chapter 17

Opening a New Dental Practice or Relocating

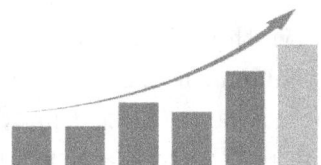

Opening a New Practice

Opening a new dental practice carries many risks. However, it is natural for dentists to finish their studies, accumulate a few years of experience, and want to open a practice in order to achieve economic and professional independence. The problem is that most dental schools do not train future dentists to open a practice and manage it from a business-marketing aspect, so at this stage, dentists are in a field that they do not know and act according to intuition only, which increases the chances of making the wrong business decisions.

Moreover, in most cases, those who study dentistry are less talented in business and marketing. If this were a strong suit for them, they probably would have gone to study business administration. Therefore, even if young dentists were to study the basics of business management at dental school, this would probably only make the problem worse rather than solve it. Over the years, I have encountered quite a few cases of dental practices that did not survive for long because the procedure of opening the practice was not done systematically or professionally, or in certain cases, the practice should not have been opened in the first place.

Needless to say, a practice's failure is not a trivial matter and usually accompanied by big debts. Here are some important principles to consider carefully before deciding to open a new practice.

1. **Are you sure you need it?** – Having a practice is not the goal but the means. Some dentists make a very good living as employees or freelancers in other

practices and perhaps they should not open a practice. Another thing is that not everyone is fit to run his or her own business. There are excellent dentists who are business owners but are such bad managers that it is better for them to work for someone else. It is better to put aside the ego that says, "I want my own practice!" As mentioned, it is best to open a practice only on the condition that the result would be better than being an employee.

2. **Financial investment** – Many new practice owners fall into this category. They invest all of their money (which is always beyond what they planned to spend) on modern furniture and equipment, panoramic photography, plasma screens, new parquets, and units – leaving no money for advertising that there is a new practice in the area. The result? There is a new, well-equipped practice, but no one knows that it exists.

   So what should be done? Well, the first step in establishing a new practice should be experimental – in the first two years, it is not worth investing too much in equipment and furniture. For example, you can use refurbished, basic furniture while investing resources mainly in bringing new patients to the practice. Only after an initial patient pool is accumulated and stable sales cycles are reached, and you decide that this is the right place for years to come, invest in the practice and upgrade it as needed.

3. **Advertising** – Just as you cannot light a barbecue without combustible material, it is impossible to build a new patient pool without a massive investment in advertising. The investment in advertising must be made over a number of months and on all channels (in accordance with the existing budget) in order to inform your surroundings of the new practice's existence and create an initial movement towards the practice. After the patient pool is built, it is possible to dilute advertising and switch to maintenance advertising. Skipping this step may create very slow growth at the practice, if at all.

4. **Building a new practice or purchasing an existing one** – It is usually preferable to purchase an existing practice rather than to set up a new one, provided you can buy the right practice at the right price. Buying an existing practice is a complex matter, mainly because of the difficulty of assessing the practice's value. "Passing the baton" from the seller to the buyer requires special attention. At the same time, a big advantage in the purchase of an existing practice is that you can start working immediately, knowing for sure what the practice does and assess how much it can do. In general, it is easier to improve an existing situation than to

build something from scratch in most cases. Working properly with the existing practice database can provide excellent initial work for the practice buyer, provided that this is a good practice with an active and loyal customer base.

5. **Business plan** – Those who skip the business plan stage take a dangerous risk. For example, you may find that expenses are much higher than you expected and enter into a cash flow crisis that will make it difficult to continue operating the practice. The business plan should include all the steps that should be carried out in the first year or two, with both pessimistic and optimistic scenarios, and be prepared for all cases. How many investors are there? Where should you advertise? What should you advertise? How much should you advertise? What other marketing actions should you take? How much does this cost? What will the practice's concept be? And so on and so forth. Of course, building a business plan should be done by a professional experienced in the dental practice field; the better the plan, the greater the chance of success.

By the way, the business plan may reveal that you do not have enough money at this stage to open a practice. Very good! It is better to wait a year or two and open a practice when you have the means to do so rather than opening too soon with a high probability of failure.

6. **Practice concept** – Will the practice focus on dental implants and be called the "Dental Implant Center" or would it be a dental center for the whole family? Will cheap or expensive rates be charged? Will it employ only specialists or general dentists? Will the practice have an arrangement with insurance agencies? And so on. You should define the practice's concept in advance: what does it offer and to whom? These questions are not simple and the answers should be included in the business plan. Of course, the practice's concept should take into account the demographic environment and all the elements that constitute the competition.

7. **Location** – The location of the new practice is of great importance. It is worth remembering that a dental practice does not have to be located on a main street, because practices are not built on passersby, however it is very important to pay attention to accessibility by public transportation and parking for patients who come in a vehicle.

8. **Partnerships** – There are cases where dentists do not feel secure enough to open a dental practice alone and therefore look for a partner. Partnership is a wonderful

thing but we need to remember that it is a complex, economic relationship, which might end with an ugly divorce. Therefore, the type of partnership must be carefully examined: who are the partners, what level of contact do you have with them, and as a rule, it is worthwhile to aspire to start alone and introduce a partner only if the need arises. Along the way, you may find that dental practice management is not necessarily a complicated matter; all you need for the first stages is to recruit a good team, an accountant, and a business-marketing consultant who understands dental practices.

9. **Goals** – Anyone who establishes a new practice must understand that they are entering a process in which the main fruits will be reaped only after a few years. The main target of the first years should be building a circle of satisfied customers who will be the practice's "ambassadors." In this context, it is important to note that at this stage the practice will usually work at a relatively low price range, to capture as many market segments as possible and bring as many customers to the practice as possible. After achieving this goal, you may move to the target of profitability, including a gradual increase in prices and a reduction in advertising and marketing.

Relocating the Dental Practice

Many dental practices consider moving to a new location at some point. There are many reasons to relocate your practice, but the main reason in most cases is, "I'll make more money at the new location." When practice owners turn to me to help them carry out the move from the marketing and business perspective, I take them back a step to the question, "Is it really right for you to move the practice at this stage? Are you more likely to earn more at the new location?"

In many cases, this reconsideration proves that business-wise it is not worthwhile to move to a new location and in the end, not only will the owner of the practice not gain more, but will probably lose. Why? Because many practice owners do not take the business and economic implications of the transition to another location into account, and work mainly in an emotional manner – "I have to leave" – and eventually regret the move. Here are five key points to consider before deciding to move to a new location.

A. **Moving costs** – Moving costs can easily amount to tens of thousands of dollars depending on the size of the practice and its number of units. It also depends on whether you will use the existing equipment or upgrade to new equipment. The practice transfer refund can take a number of years, if at all.

B. Customers do not like changes – Customers have gotten used to your practice's location. They are used to finding parking in a particular place, they go shopping before or after the visit and are used to the unique waiting room. Any change you make to the practice, especially if you move away to a significantly different geographic location, will cause some of the loyal customers not to move with you to your new practice. Losing some of your patients is losing some of your secure income and you may not be able to afford it.

C. New place, new problems – You left the previous location because you wanted to solve a problem that bothered you, say, high rent or a small waiting room. Very logical. However, remember that every place has its problems: you may suddenly discover that there is no parking space, or that there are power outages, noise from the street, and so on.

D. Larger practice, higher expenses – Many of those who move to a new practice are looking for a larger space but do not take into account the fact that the larger the practice, the higher the fixed expenses.

I know quite a few practices that moved to a larger place and succeeded in increasing their sales cycles, but at the same time also reduced profits. For example, take a two-unit practice with a monthly turnover of $150,000, which yields X per month. If that practice moves to a bigger place, let's say with four units, it will probably also have to increase spending: higher rent, adding an administrative team, etc. The same practice will have to reach a sales cycle with a monthly average of about $240,000, only to achieve the profitability of the previous practice. The result? To justify the transition financially the practice will have to attain a much higher sales cycle than at the previous practice.

E. Moving = success? Not necessarily – Here's the bottom line: when a practice fails to realize its potential, it is often because it does not work correctly and efficiently, and not because of the location or because it is a bit crowded. I have come across crowded practices that were very successful; therefore, it is reasonable to assume that even after moving to the new place there will not be a change for the better, because the practice will continue to work in the same old and problematic method. Even worse, after the move, the practice's cash flow will be short several tens of thousands (which are usually taken as a loan) that were used for the move. This may make it much more difficult financially than it was at the previous place.

Therefore, from a strategic point of view, it is worthwhile to invest primarily in improving work processes and efficiency in the existing place before moving to a new location. If the owners of the practice invest the tens of thousands they want to invest in moving to the new place (or even part of it) in marketing and promotion activities and more efficient methods of work, they will reap greater and faster rewards.

There are, of course, cases in which a move to a new location is both the right move and leads to more positive results in the end, especially when it comes to a small and successful dental practice which can no longer contain its growing pool of patients. However, as stated, the issue of the move must be examined carefully and all considerations should be weighed in order to make the right decision; in many cases staying in the same place and improving work methods is a much better solution.

If you have already decided to move to a new location, you should do this correctly and make strategic decisions: What character will the new practice have – will it be similar to the previ3ous practice or completely different? What will be the number of units? Which location is best? Is it worth buying new or used equipment? And so on. The most import thing, of course, is to inform all of your customers about the move, through all possible advertising and marketing channels, and entice them in every possible way to come to the new location for an initial appointment.

Purchase of an Active Practice and Cost Evaluation

The purchase of an active dental practice has many advantages over the establishment of a new one. When purchasing an active dental practice, there is no need to pay for the property as required in a new place (plumbing and construction it takes to run the unit, adjusting reception stations, waiting area, carpentry work, and so on).

More importantly, the biggest advantage of buying an active dental practice is the fact that you can start working from the first moment – there is an existing customer base and no need to build it from scratch. It is important to mention that building a customer base for a new dental practice, which generates reasonable sales cycles, can take many years and come at a cost of hundreds of thousands of dollars. Moreover, when you build a new practice business potential is only theoretical, but when you buy a working practice, the potential is tangible, realistic, and easier to appreciate.

For example, if the practice produces a sales turnover of $100,000 per month and a professional analysis shows that the function of the practice is mediocre (incorrect advertising, unskilled workers, etc.), it is easy to understand that the real potential of the practice is a monthly sales cycle of $150,000-200,000. On the other hand, when a practice is first opened, there is no way of knowing what future cycles will be, and everything is in the realm of forecasts and estimates only.

Evaluating the practice's worth

Let's start from the end: there is no single formula for evaluating the worth of an active practice. In the business world, there are many formulas for evaluating an active business; the problem is that the seller adopts the formula that will lead to the higher value while the buyer adopts the formula that will assess the practice at a lower value.

However, several objective factors affect the value of a business, such as supply and demand, profitability, business turnover, and equipment or real estate value. These create a certain starting point for evaluation, which will be negotiated by the seller and buyer.

Before I present the factors that affect the value of a practice, it is worth clarifying one important matter – the value of the practice consists of two main parameters: tangibles and reputation.

A. **Tangibles** refer to all the items in the practice that can be priced in an objective manner such as units, panoramic cameras, and furniture.

B. **Reputation** refers to how much the practice brand is worth, as well as its customer base, which is already much more complicated than price.

The initial stage in assessing each practice's value is the value of the tangibles. As mentioned above, this is a relatively simple and easy assessment procedure. We examine the existing equipment, assess its wear and tear, and how much it would be worth if we wanted to sell it. The tangibles mainly include the units, furniture, computerization, x-ray equipment, etc. Usually the value of the tangibles is not high, as it is not new equipment with high depreciation and wear.

As stated, the second stage of the evaluation, which examines the practice's reputation, is much more complex. However, here are some parameters to consider and which will help you evaluate the worth of the practice's reputation.

1. **Sales turnover and profitability** are undoubtedly the two most important parameters evaluating the practice. Of course, when sales and profitability are higher, the value of the practice will be higher. Here you should look at the sales cycles and the profitability of the practice compared to what is common in the dental industry.

2. **Practice potential** – Although it is important to examine how much the practice is earning today, how much it can earn is even more important; in other words, what its business potential is. In one of my consultations, I worked with a client and recommended purchasing a practice even though it lost money and even though the seller requested a relatively high price for it. The reason for the recommendation was that my analysis showed that the practice had lost money not because it was not good, but rather because it was severely mismanaged from the marketing-organizational perspective.

   My assessment was that the practice had a reasonable potential to double the sales cycle by making some strategic changes, and the reality turned out to be even better than expected – after making some strategic changes, the practice succeeded in tripling its sales within a year and turned out to be an excellent investment.

   If we had looked only at the profitability of the practice the buyer would have decided not to purchase; however, as mentioned above, what matters more is the potential and less the current situation.

3. **Examining the alternatives** – It all depends on what alternatives you have. Suppose that after examining a number of alternatives, you have two attractive options: first, an active practice with a sales turnover of $100,000 per month at a purchase price of half a million. The second option is the establishment of a new dental practice at the price of $350,000. Of course, the first option is much

more attractive, though it is more expensive. The difference between the options is $150,000 but the first includes an active customer base that generates a sales turnover of $100,000 per month, compared to the second option, which requires a large financial investment and a long time to build a customer base.

4. **Customer loyalty** – Is the practice in question one with high customer loyalty, or are most customers casual visitors who come in following advertising? This data is very important because if customers come mainly from word of mouth and there is high customer loyalty, this testifies to the strength of the practice and vice versa. If there is no loyalty to the practice, and most of the customers come in through advertising, this should be a red flag: First, why don't customers recommend the practice? Second, if customers do not recommend the practice, this means that the practice needs to invest a lot of money in advertising in order to introduce new customers, and this is not a positive situation.

   How do you check the level of customer loyalty? With two main indicators. The first is, how many customers come to the practice through word of mouth? If most customers arrive by word of mouth that means there are more recommenders, which indicates high loyalty to the practice. The second is, how many clients come in for dental hygiene treatments and periodic examinations? Customers who visit the practice every six months are evidence of loyalty to the practice. By the way, many of those who sell a practice flaunt the size of their customer pool – "I have 22,000 customers in the database" – but what matters is not how many customers there are in the database, but rather how many of them are active and loyal to the practice.

5. **Miscellaneous** – Two other parameters should be examined in order to evaluate the practice's worth.
   A. **Fixed costs** – A practice with high fixed costs such as rent or management fees is less attractive than a practice that offers low fixed costs.

   B. **Labor** – Will the existing personnel remain or should new workers be recruited? In most cases, a good employee should stay, mostly because this provides continuity for customers, and this is one of the most important things in purchasing an existing practice.

Activity after purchasing an active practice

The stage following the purchase of an active dental practice and transfer of ownership from the seller to the buyer is critical to the future success of the practice. The move should be as quick and smooth as possible for the practice's employees and of course the clients. Just like in a relay race, the baton should pass without slowing down the speed of the runners and, of course, without falling.

However, from a great deal of experience, this is a complex and sensitive process; the practice's employees, both administrative and medical, are in a state of uncertainty and fear regarding their continued employment at this stage, and full of doubts about the identity and plans of the new employer. Moreover, uncertainty and fears exist among customers as well – "We have been receiving treatment from Dr. Jones for 20 years. Who is the new dentist? Is he as good as Dr. Jones is?"

Therefore, in order for the practice's buyer to get through the first stages in the smoothest way, it is worthwhile to do the following.

1. **No revolutions!** – Since the staff is in a state of uncertainty, it is most important that the new practice owner address their fears. The last thing a new practice owner needs is a team full of fears and uncertainty, which is transferred to customers as well. Therefore, at the initial stage of receiving the practice it is worthwhile to gather all of the employees for an acquaintance meeting and tell them, "Ladies and gentlemen, everything remains the same, only better."

   It is recommended to also hold individual conversations with each employee, in order to get to know them better and identify existing problems in the practice, and primarily to reduce the uncertainty. In one of the consulting jobs I undertook in purchasing a practice, I took this recommendation a step further and implemented a small wage increase for the administrative team, which turned out to be a very successful move. Not only did the uncertainty of the workers disappear, but miraculously the motivation also increased and so did the sales turnover.

   By the way, not only the employees are in a state of uncertainty at this stage but also the practice's new owner – even more than everyone else is. Therefore, the practice owner also needs a few months in order to adjust to the new practice, and it is best to make as few revolutionary changes as possible in the first stage.

Of course, after the initial stage it is possible to perform more strategic and revolutionary moves.

2. **The transfer of the medical baton** – As mentioned, the practice's customers, who are accustomed to the medical staff after many years, are also in a state of uncertainty, and this matter must also be dealt with. The best method for making customers feel safe is to request that, as part of the practice purchase agreement, the dentist who sold the practice stay as an employee for a period, preferably about a year.

At the same time, as a first step, it is advisable to issue a letter from the dentist, who is familiar to all practice customers, which will inform them of the change in the practice's ownership. The letter should be in the following style. "Dear patient, I would like to personally inform you that ownership of the practice and medical management is transferred from me to Dr. Sierra. It is important that you know that the practice will continue to function as it has, and will continue to provide quality treatment and personal attention. Dr. Sierra is an excellent dentist, with X years of experience in dentistry, and has participated in many training programs in the areas of dental implants and rehabilitation. I will also stay here for the coming year."
Passing the baton from the previous dentist the new one will take place during this year. The veteran dentist will recommend the new dentist to the loyal customers who come to the practice: "Dr. Sierra is my heir. He's a pro and he has a golden touch. You can set your mind at ease; you will continue to receive treatments at the same level as you would with me."

The fact that the previous dentist is still at the practice, and the fact that he recommends the new dentist, will greatly increase the chances that loyal customers will continue to come to the practice and receive care with the new dentist. Of course, not all previous customers will continue to pursue care at the practice, but if the transfer is done correctly, a high percentage will. After all, the alternative is to look for a new dentist. If this is the case anyway, a dentist recommended by the old and familiar dentist is preferable.

3. **Preliminary check-up** – Moving the practice over to a new dentist is a good time to perform an intensive and thorough telemarketing campaign directed at the existing customer base, with the aim of bringing in more customers for a periodic checkup with the new dentist. For this to work, it is worthwhile to

consider offering an attractive one-time offer to customers, for example, periodic inspection plus two free x-rays plus a dental hygiene treatment, at 50% off the regular price.

This benefit should be noted at the end of the letter sent to the practice's clients (see previous section) and after the customers receive the letter by mail, telemarketers should tell customers about the new benefits and schedule them for exams and hygiene treatments.

4. **Advertising campaign** – Parallel to the work on the existing database, the new practice owner should start a campaign to attract new clients. The new customers' exams should only be performed by the new dentists so that the new customer base can start to be built around them.

Chapter 18

Dealing with Competitors

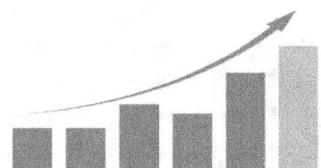

Competition for customers' hearts and pockets in the dental industry is constantly becoming fiercer. There is an explanation for this: in the last decade, the number of dentists everywhere has grown significantly. In addition, new and large dental practices are investing millions in marketing and sales promotion in order to bring in new customers to their practices, and if this is not enough, your customers always know of a few other good dentists who happen to also be located in your area.

Perhaps you will be comforted by the fact that the intensity of competition has affected every business in the market: nowadays there are a great many lawyers, accountants, architects, and insurance agents, as well as dentists. As competition intensifies, so does the need to receive tools on how to deal with it, both strategically and tactically. Paradoxically, marketing experts agree that business competition is a good thing. Of course, this is only true if you know how to handle the competition. Here are five tips to help you turn your competition from a threat into a business opportunity.

1. **Do not slander competitors** – Even though competition quickly becomes an emotional struggle, do not slander competitors. Anyone who slanders competitors is perceived by customers, at best, as insecure and helpless, and at worst, as sneaky. It is best to emphasize your strengths to your customers rather than tell them where your competitors are weak. If you really want to play down your competitors, you should actually root for them (don't exaggerate, of course).
Sound strange? Not at all; customers will conclude that you are so good that you allow yourself to speak highly of competitors. For example, you should never say to customers, "Who performed this bad treatment?" There is another reason: if

clients understand that they have chosen the wrong dentist, it will be difficult for them to choose you because they will be afraid of making another bad decision.

2. **Your competitor's advantage is also their disadvantage** – Is your competitor large? They are probably weak when it comes to personal interactions. Are your competitors veterans? They are probably outdated and not innovative. Like in the ancient Chinese martial arts law, it is recommended to use the opponent's strength against them. For example, the advantage of size, when it comes to public practices, can also be their weak point. You can always tell clients, "Yes, you can undergo the treatment at a public practice and save some money, but what if you have a problem in a year or two? Will the dentist who cared for you still be there to take care of you?" Or, you can always say to customers who receive a very cheap treatment plan offer from another practice, "Mr. Smith, the cheapest is usually expensive in the long run. As in everything in life, there is a direct connection between quality and price."

3. **Define who your direct competitors are** – The direct competitor of a specialist is a specialist, rather than a general dentist. The direct competitor of a private practice is a private dental practice, not a public one. Always be sure to ask the clients to make a fair comparison: "Mr. Smith, we should compare apples to apples and not to pears. A private practice is not a public practice with all that entails."

4. **Don't try to be better than your competitor** – Be different! In many cases, those who try to attack competitors by using the "better" strategy end the battle bruised and with a big hole their pocket. Therefore, it is usually recommended to use the differentiation strategy; is your direct competitor working at low prices? Raise your prices and you will be perceived as providing a higher quality of care.

5. **"Know your enemy!"** – The better you get to know your competitors, the better you can deal with them. In fact, you will not be able to conduct effective negotiations with your customers if you don't have the data about what your competitors offer. Therefore, you should send "undercover clients" periodically to find out what prices are charged at competing practices, what's new in their waiting room, and how they deal with customers. There may be things you can adopt in your practice, or alternatively, if you encounter negative elements, you can make sure they do not happen at your practice.

Chapter 19

Aesthetic Treatments

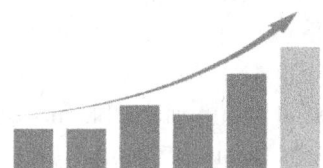

In recent years, more and more dentists have begun to discover the business potential inherent in facial aesthetic treatments such as Botox injections, wrinkle filling, etc. And no wonder – the profit is high, the work is easy, and even more enjoyable than traditional dental treatments. Additionally, the immediate aesthetic results of these treatments lead to satisfaction and happiness for both dentists and clients.

However, not everything is so rosy. Dental practices that don't combine the aesthetic treatments correctly with the traditional treatments cause confusion in the positioning of the practice. The result? Confusing positioning leads clients to flee from the familiar treatments and most of all from transplants and oral rehabilitation, which causes financial damage to the practice.

One of the most basic rules in marketing is, "Both this and that equals neither." Specialization in one specific field leads professionals to become experts in their field and grants them credit points with customers. Just as in the case of specialists, patients will feel more comfortable to undergo root canal treatment at the root canal specialist.

However, this rule also works the other way around – if the professional deals with a large number of areas, his or her professional image will decrease. If the professional does both this and that, they are perceived as being mediocre in all of the areas.

So, what happens to clients who need dental implants and full-mouth rehabilitation, and see that the dental practice also offers Botox and wrinkle filling, compared to customers who go to a practice that only deals with dental implants and even calls itself "The Implant Center"? Where will they feel more comfortable to undergo this complex treatment? At the all-in-one practice or the one that specializes in dental implants and oral rehabilitation? The second option is the answer, of course.

Thus, the practice gains quick and easy revenues with high profit margins from the aesthetic treatments, but on the other hand, loses clients for full oral rehab.

Moreover, with all due respect to the profitability of aesthetic treatments, the big money is actually found in dental implants and full oral rehabilitation.

So what should be done? First, it is important that any dentist who also does aesthetic treatments understands the positioning problem that may arise due to combining these treatments. The way to solve this is quite simple: dental practices should not give up on these treatments, but in order to solve the positioning problem, they should separate dental treatments from aesthetic treatments.

For example, the practice's advertising should not mention both types of treatments together, so as not to create confusion. Want to promote aesthetics on Facebook? No problem; open up a separate business page. Want to advertise in the local press? No problem; publish a separate ad.

This should be done for all types of advertising. The issue of investing in advertising and marketing should also be considered. I once encountered a practice that has a rotation: a week of advertising for dental work and a week of advertising for aesthetics. When we examined what percentage of sales came from aesthetics out of the total turnover, we found that it was only 8%.

Of course, this is not financially logical – an advertising budget cannot be divided 50-50 between dentistry and aesthetic treatments when the percentage of sales is 8:92 in favor of dentistry. There must be a direct connection between advertising investment and contribution to the practice's income. So how do you still market aesthetic treatments? Mainly through marketing in the course of the dentist's personal interaction with the patient, while they are sitting in the chair. For example: "Ms. Green, in addition to the aesthetic treatment we performed on your front teeth, and because your lips are quite narrow, I think we can improve your smile with this and that treatment," or a conversation about wrinkles along the lines of, "Did you know that you could easily hide this wrinkle?"

In conclusion, aesthetic treatment is a good field that can certainly be complementary to dentistry, so you should incorporate it into a dental practice. It is only a supplementary field and accordingly must be adjusted to the main activity of the practice so as not to harm your work.

PART SIX

MISCELLANEOUS

Chapter 20

Dealing with Demanding Customers

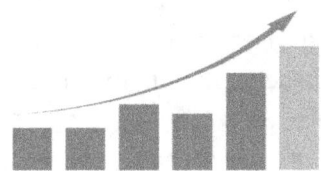

I received an urgent call one day from the manager of a dental practice I had consulted. "I can't deal with this client; he drives me crazy. You have to help me. How should I deal with this?" she asked desperately. "Please look at the client's treatment plan," I told her. "Now, how much money is he worth to the practice?" The manager did the short calculation and replied, "He just started the treatment, and the plan is worth $27,000."

"Okay," I replied. "Now call the owners and ask if they are willing to give up $27,000. If so, let the client go! If not, drink some cold water, be patient, and do everything in your power to treat him to his satisfaction." About half an hour later, the manager called again and informed me that, "That everything had been settled with the client and all is well."

You're probably familiar with the client that the manager encountered – he asks much too many questions, clings to details, only has complaints, is problematic when it comes to payment, and is always sure that he is right and you are wrong. Nice to meet you, Mr. Demanding! In fact, about 15% of your customers are demanding to some extent. If it's any comfort then statistically, all businesses have a similar percentage of demanding customers. The same customers bother everyone, not just you. They're just like that. I would not have devoted a full chapter to demanding customers if it were not 15%! Even though the thing you most want to do is ask those customers to leave and close the door behind them, you do not have the luxury of giving up 15% of your customers. This is such a high percentage that it may make the difference between a profitable practice and an unprofitable one. Because we have no way to change the nature of these customers, we should know how to deal with them so that we do not lose them.

Here are some tips to help you and your practice staff deal with demanding customers. But first, relax! Many service providers fail in their dealings with demanding customers.

1. **They see this as a personal matter** ("How dare he talk to me like that?") – If the customer's demands have succeeded in driving you crazy and you are beginning to think and respond from your gut and not from your head, you've lost. Therefore, although it is difficult, you have to go about this in a cool and intelligent manner. In most cases, the customer has nothing against Delia. In such situations, Delia should detach emotionally and conduct herself in front of them as the practice's representative.

2. **I understand you, Mr. Right** – If someone is preparing for a fight and, to his surprise, you actually reach out to him, in most cases he will shake your hand and feel embarrassed. The same strategy should be implemented with demanding customers. Is the customer yelling? Speak softly. Is he complaining about a delay? Instead of saying that the delay is not your responsibility, be empathic, tell him you understand his anger, stand by him, and show him that you understand. For example, "I know what you mean, Mr. Right," or, "I'm very sorry for the delay; I understand how much this is disrupting your plans." You might be surprised how quickly he will relax.

3. **Change the tune** – If you think of these clients as demanding or nagging, your conduct towards them will be the same. In this situation, you can rest assured that the problem will not be resolved and that the course of events will develop in a negative direction and strengthen the clients' antagonism towards you and the practice.

So, start the process positively. Ask yourself, "Maybe it really is a failure of ours? Is the client's anger justified?" In addition, try to think about how you would react if you were in their place. Yes, you too get angry and sometimes even shout when there is a big gap between what you expect and what you receive.

Here's a good example. In one of the consultations I performed, the dentist said to me, as he glanced at the appointment book, "The most annoying customer you have ever seen is about to walk in. He does not stop complaining, moaning, and he has questions from here to Alaska." I replied, "Let's try an exercise: go out to the waiting room, hug him, ask him how he is and how his family is doing, and watch him become your most easy-going customer."

The dentist did so, and so it was – the client did not make a peep; he sat calmly and did not have one complaint during the entire treatment. When the dentist asked me why, I explained the obvious to him: "Because you thought he was a nuisance, you treated him as such; so you received an annoying client. This time you treated him as a kind and gentle man and thereby removed every desire or motivation he had to be a nuisance." Have you ever heard of a prophecy fulfilling itself?

4. **How much will this cost us?** – Studies show that, on average, dissatisfied customers tell about 12 acquaintances about their experience. Imagine what happens when it comes to demanding clients, who in many cases are also loud: we have negative publicity of the worst kind, with the potential for causing enormous financial damage to the practice. Therefore, if you direct the whole staff to put their egos aside and think about the customers (and their acquaintances) in economic terms, you will suddenly find that they are more tolerant – even more so if you can make them understand that losing customers could lead to them losing their jobs.

5. **Demanding clients = good customers** – You will be surprised, but it is precisely those demanding customers who complain, call often, and cause difficulty, who are actually good clients. The customers' claims indicate that they are involved and interested in contact with the practice. If they did not care, they would be indifferent and leave without drama, as many customers do. In addition, if you know how to deal with them, they will not leave you. Therefore, it is worth seeing the demanding clients as an opportunity rather than a threat.

6. **No chemistry? Replace the service or sales representative** – A client who raises his or her voice to Iris may develop a good relationship with Delia. So if you do not have chemistry with demanding clients and you see that you are on a collision course, have someone who will be able to find something in common with him deal with him or her.

7. **Determination and sensitivity** – If you have completed all the previous sections but to no avail, it's a sign that you're dealing with a mega-demanding customer. This represents less than 1% of customers; they demand so many resources and energy from the practice that any economic benefit that might be produced in this case is much lower than the benefit. In such a situation, it is worthwhile and even recommended to initiate a proactive disengagement from client – with determination, but also with sensitivity.

Chapter 21

Business Conduct during the Holidays

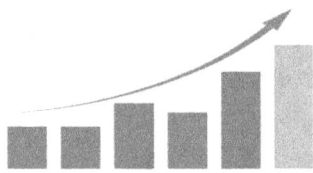

Holidays and summer vacations are problematic for dental practices and no wonder; people like to postpone dental treatments and the holidays serve as an excellent excuse for this ("We'll be in touch after the holidays"). This could create a significant drop in practice revenues.

So what can be done? Probably not sitting idly by. You can minimize damage before a holiday period by using the foot-in-the-door sales tactic.

The foot-in-the-door marketing tactic, which has been researched scientifically, claims that consent to a small part of a transaction or even a small step in the transaction process significantly increases the chances of reaching the overall closing of the transaction. Therefore, when clients say, "We'll talk after the holidays," they must be respected but you must also insist on a small step to be done now (a small filling, plaque removal, etc.), which will increase the chances of closing the big deal – after the holidays, of course.

How do you do this? Suggest that the client start with a dental hygiene treatment and another small treatment, for example, "Mr. Smith, let's start with a dental hygiene treatment to stop the inflammation, and we'll perform a filling in tooth X so that you do not experience food compression. After the holidays, we will discuss the implant proposal for the lower jaw." Another example: "Mr. Smith, no problem, we'll talk after the holiday. Let's just start with a dental hygiene treatment; you must do this anyway, regardless of the treatment plan." Or, "Let's take measurements so that we will not be delayed after the holidays when you want to start treatment," and so on.

You should even make it clear to the customer that this is not binding, for example:

"Mr. Smith, even if you decide not to go through with the whole plan in the end, you need to remove plaque in any case, in order to treat the inflammation. You should do this now with our excellent hygienist, so that after the holiday you can continue with whatever part of the plan you choose." As stated, once the customer starts a treatment, even the smallest one, this will significantly increase the chance that they will continue the treatment at the practice.

Chapter 22

The Little Things That Make a Big Difference

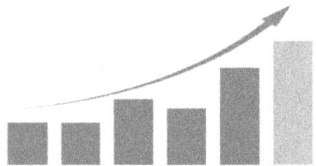

"Marketing is in the details," goes the famous phrase. Everyone knows the big things; you will only succeed if you are better at the little things.

Here are eight small things that can make a big difference at your dental practice.

1. **How can I help you today?** – When customers arrive for an exam and settle into the chair, ask them, "How can I help you today?" Subconsciously, the additional word 'today' may lead clients to start a treatment, even a small one, today.

2. **Yes or yes?** – Don't ask customers questions with 'yes or no' answers. Why? Because you are increasing the likelihood that they will say 'no'! Therefore, don't ask, "Do you want to start treatment?" but rather, "When is it convenient for you to undergo treatments, in the morning or in the evening?" The same way that street food vendors don't ask, "Do you want a drink?" but, "What will you have, Coke or orange soda?"

3. **Plaque Removal** – Seventy dollars for a "cleaning" is a high price. However, the same amount for "plaque removal" is another matter. In addition, cleaning is only an aesthetic matter while a removal is both medical and aesthetic, and therefore the practice staff should only use the term "removal."

4. **A quote?** – A quote is usually received from renovators and mechanics, while the dentist offers a "treatment plan proposal." It sounds medical and professional and therefore make it a rule for your practice: Do not use the word 'quote.'

5. **Exactly two days** – A customer who received a treatment plan offer and left the matter with, "Let me think about it," should receive a phone call from the

receptionist or practice manager after exactly two days! Why two days? Because that's the amount of time in which customers think they will receive additional offers from other practices, but they do not find the time to do this – and therefore, this is just the time to reel them back in.

6. **Express positivity** – Use only positive expressions. Negative phrases create negative energy that does not contribute to the atmosphere and performance of the practice. So don't say, "impossible" or "can't" – you can say the same thing only positively. For example, if a customer asks, "Is there an appointment on Sunday?" instead of saying "No," it is possible to tell them, "There's an appointment on Tuesday." It is the same answer but phrased positively.

7. **"Dr. Jones asked to see you"** – Want to increase the effectiveness of RE-CALLS? Don't use an assembly line style sentence such as, "It's been six months and we wanted to schedule a periodical checkup." Instead, tell clients, "Six months ago we performed treatments X, Y, and Z, and Dr. Jones went over your chart and asked that you come in to make sure everything is okay." If the dentist asks for this, and there is reference to the specific treatment undergone by the client, it is very likely that the customers will feel obligated to come in.

8. **What is his name?** – Why don't you use a nametag for yourself and the entire practice staff? It is easier for customers to communicate with people whose names they know and connect with them. By the way, don't assume that customers remember your name and the names of the other staff. On the other hand, you can be sure that they feel uncomfortable asking. Therefore, it is important that each member of the practice staff have a tag with their name on the left pocket of their uniform.

This book is devoted with great love
To my father,
Yosef Asulin – may he rest in peace
To my mother,
Zohara Asulin – may she rest in peace

To my children,
Romi, Yonatan, and Amit – my pride and joy
To my dear wife, Tali
And to my dear brothers and sisters.

Your Practice Can Earn More!

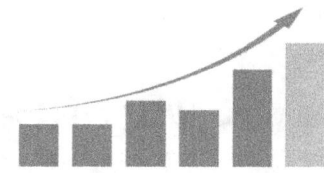

The Dental Practice Business Solutions Company offers you a variety of unique services and professional marketing counseling and support. My services will help you improve sales performance and profitability at your dental practice both in the short and long term.

We offer:
- Marketing consulting and support, in order to increase practice sales and profitability.
- Business analysis, in order to examine the practice's function.
- Examining feasibility when opening a new practice or moving to a new one.
- Drafting business plans for setting up a new practice.
- Seminars and lectures on the management and marketing of dental practices.

Over the years we have consulted hundreds of dental practices around the world, and thanks to my extensive experience, have the ability to pinpoint the problems preventing your practice from realizing its potential, and offer solutions which will lead the practice to success and profitability within a relatively short time.

We specialize not only in building the most effective business plan for your dental practice but in motivating the practice staff to implement the plan built for the practice. Over the years, we have developed unique methods for managing and marketing dental practices that achieve the best results. Implementing my management and marketing methods at your dental practice can improve your practice's business reality significantly and quickly.

The counseling and support plan are individually fashioned for each practice according to its unique needs. You are welcome to contact us for more information and find out which of my consulting and marketing support plans are suitable for you and your practice.

Contact Us: +972-77-710-0460

www.dentalmarketing.co.il